Praise for *Contraception and Catholicism*

"*Contraception and Catholicism: What the Church Teaches and Why* is a much-needed resource that offers clarity and understanding for one of the Church's most misunderstood teachings. In this volume, Dr. Angela Franks gives us an intelligent, calm, and thoughtful response to the toughest questions concerning the Church's teachings on birth control. I have enjoyed reading this book, and I encourage anyone who has questions or doubts about the Church's teaching to sit down and read this volume. Dr. Franks writes about sexual ethics in a way that engages and even entertains. Most importantly, however, her arguments and examples challenge all of us to deeper conversion and holiness in Christ. The Church's teaching on contraception is an invitation for all of us to embrace God's will, which will bring us true happiness and peace. *Contraception and Catholicism* will be a rich resource for men and women of all ages who seek an ever-deeper appreciation for the gift of human sexuality and for the treasure of the Church's teaching on sexual ethics. It's a great example of a new style of apologetics, one which engages the mind and heart and helps us to articulate our Christian beliefs, especially those that are often misunderstood or ignored."

— Cardinal Seán O'Malley, OFM Cap.,
Archbishop of Boston

"If you have ever thoug~~ht the Church's t~~ch~~ed~~ d
birth control methods ~~w~~ g
with reality, I dare you t d

for a renewed sex life. In *Contraception and Catholicism: What the Church Teaches and Why*, Angela Franks, PhD, offers reasoned explanations for why the Church is not a killjoy when it comes to sexual love. Plus, this book offers compelling evidence for why contraception is rooted in fear that slowly destroys loving relationships between men and women by demonizing human fertility and the female body in particular. Highly recommended."

— Pat Gohn, Author, *Blessed, Beautiful, and Bodacious: Celebrating the Gift of Catholic Womanhood*

"Dr. Franks' explanation of the Church's teaching on contraception is revolutionary. She appeals to nature, reality, and common sense—all of which make her argument incredibly persuasive and fun to read. This book is a must-read for all young men and women who truly desire to know the meaning and purpose of sex."

— Katie Elrod, contributor to *Women, Sex, and the Church: A Case for Catholic Teaching* and presenter on natural fertility treatment

"In 1968, Pope Paul VI was a prophet among us who tried to prevent heartache and social breakdown. We didn't listen. Angela Franks helps us pick up the pieces and to begin again, where we are. *Contraception and Catholicism: What the Church Teaches and Why* is an essential primer in our ongoing, much-needed, post-sexual-revolution renewal."

— Kathryn Jean Lopez, director, Catholic Voices USA; award-winning syndicated columnist

Contraception
and Catholicism

Contraception and Catholicism

What the Church Teaches and Why

Angela Franks, PhD

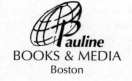

Pauline
BOOKS & MEDIA
Boston

Library of Congress Cataloging-in-Publication Data

Franks, Angela, 1971-
    Contraception and Catholicism : what the church teaches and why /
Angela Franks, PhD.
        pages cm
    ISBN-13: 978-0-8198-1638-2
    ISBN-10: 0-8198-1638-8
    1. Contraception--Religious aspects--Catholic Church. I. Title.
    HQ766.3.F73 2013
    241'.66--dc23
                                        2013020427

The Scripture quotations contained herein are from the *New Revised Standard Version Bible: Catholic Edition,* copyright © 1989, 1993, Division of Christian Education of the National Council of the Churches of Christ in the United States of America. Used by permission. All rights reserved.

Excerpts from the English translation of the *Catechism of the Catholic Church* for use in the United States of America, copyright © 1994, United States Catholic Conference, Inc. —Libreria Editrice Vaticana. Used with permission.

Cover design by Rosana Usselmann

Cover photo by © istockphoto.com/ Yuri_Arcurs

Published by Pauline Books & Media, 50 Saint Pauls Avenue, Boston, MA 02130-3491. www.pauline.org

Printed in the U.S.A.

Pauline Books & Media is the publishing house of the Daughters of St. Paul, an international congregation of women religious serving the Church with the communications media.

1 2 3 4 5 6 7 8 9   17 16 15 14 13

Contents

CHAPTER ONE

Catholic Teaching on Contraception: A Hard Pill to Swallow?

The Church makes many countercultural appeals, but there is no tougher sell than her teaching on contraception. A majority of Catholics in North America do not understand or accept the Church's claim that deliberately sterilizing the sexual act is never good for those involved. Why? Why do we find ourselves feeling we absolutely must have recourse to contraception? How did we receive this social script?

The objections to Church teaching on this point are so deeply internalized that it might be hard to articulate them. People *feel* these objections as much as they think them. But when those feelings are put into words, the words you will hear most often are usually "freedom" and "control." *Birth control* promises *personal control*: the freedom to control fertility in order to have a career, a sex life free from fear, a horizon not hemmed in by the burdens of unwanted children but open to anything one wants to achieve.

I understand where those objections are coming from—because I was one of those Catholics. As a young Catholic, I was always an engaged and curious believer, but the one point I could not comprehend was why the Church said what she did on the subject of contraception. In fact, I remember an exchange with friends as a teenager. When asked if I really agreed with *everything* the Church taught, I responded confidently, "Yes, I do." But then I had to add, "Well, maybe not the teaching about birth control." One of my friends immediately exclaimed: "Good girl!"

Indeed, the reaction was so positive that I began to be a little suspicious. Clearly, I was not staking out a countercultural position. Saying "no" to the Church on this issue was not a brave stance against the dominant paradigm. Rather, saying "no" *was* the dominant paradigm. The worldly approval I received was so contrary to what I usually encountered when expressing Church teaching on tough topics that the experience began to fester a little. I kept turning it over in my mind. The broader culture is not very healthy when it comes to sexual matters. Could it really be trusted on contraception?

As I mulled over the incident, I could not escape the dawning recognition that a panicky fear of the alternatives underlies the eager acceptance of the dominant worldview. Ridicule of Church teaching is a blustery distraction from our collective death grip on our birth control pills. Support for contraception is usually framed in positive terms, about what we can achieve and gain from birth control. But the question that should make us think even more is the negative one: what are we fleeing from? In other words, what are we all so afraid of?

Briefly, the answer is "the future." We fear what our personal futures would look like without contraception. We might allow God into every other part of our lives, but two things in particular tend to be the last bastions we defend as our own private kingdoms: money and sex. And both are about our future. Will I have enough money to do the things I want to do and to buy the things I think I need? Closely connected is sex, that is, what I do with my body and with my heart. Will I be able to live the way I want without being burdened with responsibilities that I think I cannot manage? *Will I be happy?*

In fact, our struggles over trusting God with our money and with our sex lives are proxy battles for the real war in our soul: How much do I trust that God's plan will make me happy? Will I obtain happiness by managing everything just right? Or will I find it by wholly entrusting my life to God, playing out the adventure that is the Father's plan of loving goodness precisely tailored for me? If true flourishing comes from trusting in God's plan alone, then happiness cannot be found in defining for myself what reality should be. Happiness will be found instead in being receptive to the reality that is already there, in the loving wisdom of God. Anything else is living an illusion, and illusions never make us happy.

Thus, when the Church teaches that sex *means* both love and life, both *unity* and *procreation*, she is not forcing an antiquated worldview on our intimate relationships. Rather, she is revealing the reality that is already there. Whether it is convenient or not, sex has certain contours: emotionally it bonds the two people who engage in it (even if we don't want it to), and biologically it is an evolutionary mechanism aimed at the conception of children (even if we don't want it to). If we live our sexual lives fighting these realities, we set ourselves up for frustration and unhappiness. If we are open to these realities, we find the building blocks for a healthy and intelligent sexual life.

This book will probe these ideas further. Is it really possible to live in accordance with Catholic sexual teaching? What does that life look like? What is the world offering instead, and is it really such a great deal? How can a person who has been contracepting learn to live differently? And how can this most difficult teaching be explained to others who cannot comprehend it?

I hope that reading this book is as much a spiritual as an intellectual journey. It should be an opportunity to come to a deeper conversion to the wise and loving will of God the Father in our lives. In the end, the Church's teaching on birth control is a call to surrender to *God's* control—or, rather, to his providential care—to move from fear to trust, and hence to an embrace of the happiness that only comes through receiving what our gracious and loving Father has in store for us. "What no eye has seen, nor ear heard, nor the human heart conceived, what God has prepared for those who love him" (1 Cor 2:9). The Church's teaching on contraception is a call to embrace a happiness that is infinitely greater than what we can piece together from the shreds of our own plans.

CHAPTER TWO

What People Think the Church Says

The popular mind is littered with caricatures of what the Catholic Church says about birth control. These distortions tend to circle around a couple of charges: misogyny and medievalism.

For example, a columnist for a magazine states categorically, "The Church hierarchy's objection to birth control is medieval and barbaric." He asserts that Catholics should raise some "hell with their own Church over a policy that's caused incalculable pain and misery for millions of women around the globe."[1] "Pain and misery" here refers to the epidemic of HIV/AIDS infection in Africa and elsewhere. If the Catholic Church would only allow the poor to use condoms, the argument goes, many would have been protected from the scourge of disease.

It is not only commentators looking in from the outside who take issue with Catholic teaching. Some theologians are in the vanguard of opposition to this doctrine. One such theologian, Daniel Maguire, has been agitating on this issue since the 1960s. He recently provided the following genealogy of the Church's position: "A culture that looks on women as sources of evil like Pandora and Eve is going to have trouble justifying having sex with them and may conclude that only reproduction could justify sexual collusion with women. That is exactly what happened in Christianity."[2]

Less fantastical intellectuals in the last several decades have made a case for changing Church teaching to allow contraceptive use. Before Pope Paul VI rearticulated Church teaching on contraception in his 1968 encyclical, *Humanae Vitae*, he convened an advisory committee to prepare a report on the issue of birth control. Such committees are a normal part of Vatican life, and they are meant to operate silently under the radar and disappear when the pope thanks them for their work and takes or leaves it. This particular committee, however, leaked its report to the media. The "Majority Report" revealed that a majority of the theologians and experts on the committee had recommended a reversal in Church teaching. The leaked paper set up an expectation in the Catholic world that its recommendations would be accepted. This attempt to pressure the pope into acquiescing was unsuccessful, but the larger strategy worked: theologians set themselves up as an alternate teaching authority within the Church and were empowered to engage in open war on Church teaching.

What did the Majority Report argue? It claimed that certain factors allowed a reconsideration of Church teaching. These factors included

> social changes in matrimony and the family, especially in the role of the woman; lowering of the infant mortality rate; new bodies of knowledge in biology, psychology, sexuality, and demography; a changed estimation of the value and meaning of human sexuality and of conjugal relations; most of all, a better grasp of the duty of man to humanize and to bring to greater perfection for the life of man what is given in nature.[3]

So the committee advised that the most important factor in marital sexuality should be the overall intent of a married couple to be open to life:

> Therefore the morality of sexual acts between married people takes its meaning first of all and specifically

from the ordering of their actions in a fruitful married life, that is, one which is practiced with responsible, generous, and prudent parenthood. It does not then depend upon the direct fecundity of each and every particular act.[4]

In other words, as long as the couple is open to being parents in an *overall* sense, individual sexual acts can be contracepted.

Catholics need to understand the impact that theologians such as Daniel Maguire and the authors of the Majority Report have had upon the average Catholic. It is unlikely that Maguire and similar thinkers have directly shaped the thought-worlds of most laypeople (that is, Catholics who are not priests or professed religious), since the laity usually do not read theology in their spare time. But theologians train priests in seminaries, and they teach Catholic school teachers, parish staff, and other lay leaders. Bad theology as well as good trickles down to the laity through parishes, Catholic schools, and Catholic universities. If the majority of theologians go astray, most Catholics will eventually be led into error. And since some theologians have set themselves up as authorities rivaling the popes, until fairly recently it was difficult for the non-professional to be able to discern truth from error.

The theological trickle-down effect has affected an enormous swath of Catholics. Whatever the correct statistic, at least a large majority of adult Catholics are using birth control. One of these, a female college student, writes, "Even though the official Catholic Church teaches against contraceptives, I do not feel immoral using them. They've allowed me to live my life without the fear of unwanted pregnancies or deadly diseases."[5] Here are encapsulated many of the ideologies of our time: a morality dictated by feeling; the assumed inevitability of extramarital sexual activity as necessary for human fulfillment; and the unconsidered idea that contraception is a magic cure for unwanted pregnancy and disease. This book will explore the viability of these ideas. In the next chapter, I will propose that living our lives grounded in *reality* rather than in our *emotional reactions to reality* is the only way to an authentically happy life, a life of intelligence and true love.

CHAPTER THREE

What the Church Actually Says

Clarity about contraception requires a renewed effort to think critically. The rest of this book will flesh out the Church's teaching and critique the claims for contraception.

Be attentive to reality: this is the fundamental appeal the Church makes in all her teaching, especially when it comes to contraception. What is the reality of sex, of relationships, of love and intimacy, of family? I am not talking about what passes as "reality" today—certainly not the "reality" of the ironically named reality TV. I do not mean the "reality" that we construct and pretend is the real thing. And I do not mean the "reality" that has already been constructed by society and that we consume uncritically. Are a feverish child's hallucinations real? They are experiences, certainly, but do these experiences harmonize with the actual structures and processes of the world? Or do they distort the fabric of the real?

One might argue, "Adults freely making sexual decisions are autonomous agents, and they can construct their own reality. Who are you to say they can't?" Yet how autonomous are we adults, really? Just as the sick child's imagination becomes passively subject to the power of the illness, so too do we let our imaginations fall hostage to the febrile forces of the dominant culture. A quick glance at the portrayal of sex in music videos, sitcoms, and movies (try this with the sound off) reveals a definite parody of reality. All the scenes are scripted, rehearsed, filmed with lighting, and edited with background music and sound effects, including the few that are true to the feel and rhythm of the real. But pay particular attention to the homogenized representation of sexuality. Where is the authenticity? If you stop to think about what you are seeing, does it have even the minimum elements of dramatic plausibility? And most of us simply adapt our views of sex from what we passively consume from various media. It is a banquet of unreality. No wonder we are so hungry.

So when the Church reminds us of the need to *be attentive to reality*, this can't mean "pay attention to what lots of other people are doing," or "imitate what you see on TV," or (worst of all) "never let an itchy desire go unscratched." We have to recognize that reality is something to be discovered, not manufactured. A more philosophical way of speaking about it is to say that reality is *given*, not invented by us.

It is tempting to try to create our own world. Isn't that a big part of the appeal of virtual identities, which promise to recreate ourselves from nothing? My desires become the measure of all things. I will have the lifestyle I want, no matter what. Consumerism and relativism mean never having to say you're sorry. We become absolute masters of our tiny corner of the universe.

The alternative to this egoistic way of personal existence is the way of gratitude. Instead of shaping reality according to idiosyncratic whim, the grateful person tries to discern what has already been given in reality. When it comes to intimacy, sex, and contraception, this means that, instead of treating sex as an arbitrary instrument of self-gratification (the egoist), the grateful person tries to understand the meaning that is to be found in sex before arriving on the scene. When we unwrap the gift that is sex, what do we find?

After a few generations of being told that liberation means living like sexual egoists, it is really hard for us to live in a grateful receptivity to reality. The social avenues leading out of the prison of the self have long since been blockaded. Could sex possibly have a *purpose*, other than deliciously scratching that urgent sexual itch? Younger generations have been told for years in sex education that genital pleasure is simply a matter of making *me* feel good, nothing more.

Think how absurd it would be if we approached other areas of our lives like this. Take driving, for example. What if cars simply existed to satisfy my automotive urges, and to provide opportunities to experience the sheer pleasure of driving? We would get the ridiculous picture of the entire automotive industry existing so that people could . . . what? Drive around in circles in a field or on solitary racecar tracks? No doubt cars can be a lot of fun to drive, but that pleasure is not the *point* of driving. Rather, it is the *by-product* of driving. The *point* of an automobile is more pedestrian (if you will pardon the mixed metaphor). The purpose is to get you from point A to point B. If it happens to be a lot of fun in the process, all the better, but you do not get the by-product without the purpose. (Even car races and country drives depend on the reality of the primary purpose.)

The example of eating is even easier to understand. Why do we eat? Because it is pleasurable? Not really. If a person hasn't eaten for two days and then is presented with something that is not very enjoyable to eat, like stale bread, she is not going to say, "Thanks, but I'll hold off for another day or two. That is not enjoyable enough for me to eat." No, we eat because we need to nourish ourselves. Nourishment is the *purpose*. Pleasure is the *by-product*. An evolutionary biologist might say that we enjoy eating so that we will do it, so that the race will survive. The by-product of pleasure serves the purpose of nourishment.

So it is with sex. The very real (and good) by-product that is sexual pleasure serves the purpose of sex. Evolutionary biologists have something to say here as well. If we ask them why most of the animal world features sex, they will tell you it is for *reproduction*. For more complex species, why is it pleasurable (the by-product)? For the *purpose* of reproduction.

I was once in a moral theology class with a group of seminarians. One raised his hand and queried exasperatedly, "Why did God make sex so pleasurable if the pleasure causes so many problems?" The professor sighed, rolled his eyes, and enunciated slowly, "Because if sex . . . were . . . like . . . *calculus* . . . the race would have died out long ago!" Because sex is pleasurable, we humans want to do it. And because we want to do it, we make little humans. And little humans continue the species.

All this language of biology might seem very crass. It certainly doesn't sound like the love songs that have been sung for centuries. Where's the romance? Where's the three-hankie chick-flick movie plot? Where's the *love*?

Well, love is part of the picture too, as we'll see. But I started with the biology because I want to prevent the common misconception that you love with some ghostly part of yourself, maybe called the *real you* (or your *soul*, if you are religious), and have sex with the bodily part of yourself, and the two can somehow be neatly separated. Here's a reality check: *you* are an animal. You are not *only* an animal. You are also rational (I'll get to that in a minute). But you are still an animal. You are embodied, with a body that was conceived and is nourished and one day will die, just like that of any other animal. And animals reproduce through sex. Your reproductive system is meant for, well, reproducing, just as much as your dog's reproductive system is meant for reproducing. That is its purpose.

"But," you say, "I've seen my dog in heat, and that is most certainly *not* what human sex is about. Dogs *have* to have sex. But humans are free, and their sex has meaning. Are you saying humans are just like dogs in heat?"

No, I am not saying that, although a lot of other people say that (Hugh Hefner, for example). Here is where the rationality of humans comes in. We are *rational* animals. What does that mean? It doesn't mean that we are unemotional robots. It means that, unlike Fido, we *know* and—here's that word!—*love*. In addition to our animal bodies, we also have intellects and free wills, which are meant to be used for knowing and loving each other and God.

In saying that human beings are "spiritual," philosophy is referring to this capacity for knowing and loving. Being spiritual does not mean that we like new age music and incense. It means that we have the power to do what is above the physical, although we have to use our bodily organs to do it. When we love someone, hearts don't actually appear over our heads, despite the cartoons. Love is spiritual, transcending space and time. Yet we cannot express love without our bodies; we can't even have a conversation with a friend we love without our bodies. Even more so, human sex is *both* physical and spiritual.

From this background, we can understand what the Church is getting at when she says that sex means both "procreation" and "union," as Pope Paul VI says in paragraph twelve of his encyclical *Humanae Vitae*. On the one hand, the reproductive system is oriented to reproduction: that's *procreation*. On the other hand, the entire experience of human sexuality is meant to unite two people not just physically but also spiritually: that's *unity*. Dr. Janet Smith calls these two aspects of human sexuality "babies and bonding." [1]

"Wait a minute," you might object. "How can you say that part of the *meaning* and *purpose* of sex is procreation? What about infertile couples—can't they have sex?" Let's return to our car analogy: We have ascertained that cars have a purpose, which is to get you from point A to point B. Sadly, some cars don't achieve that purpose. They don't run. I'm not a car person, but I gather this problem can be due to, say, a faulty carburetor. Suppose my hatchback has this affliction and does not run; does this mean that cars in general no longer have the purpose to get us from point A to point B? Well, no, it just means that my particular car is not capable of fulfilling its purpose until it is fixed. So, too, with couples suffering from infertility. For any number of reasons, tragically, one or both of their reproductive systems cannot achieve the end of procreation. But that doesn't mean that reproductive systems in general are not oriented to reproduction.

(NaProTECHNOLOGY, an ethical way to treat infertility issues, gives some reasons for hope when facing the tragedy of infertility.)[2]

We cannot change the purpose of cars from transportation to nourishment, for example, just because we think it might be cool to eat our cars instead of driving them. Whatever our *intention*, reality has its own rules that transcend what goes on between our ears. Likewise, we cannot change the nature of sex from being about babies and bonding to being about pleasure-as-an-end just because we think it might be fun to enjoy sexual pleasure without any possibility of kids, or because we'd like to hook up with a stranger and avoid any emotional entanglements thereafter. Insisting that pleasure is the purpose of eating rather than its by-product makes us fat and unhealthy. Insisting that pleasure is the purpose of sex rather than its by-product makes us sexually gluttonous and unhealthy—and deeply unhappy.

Living like egoists doesn't work: reality always pushes back. The only solution is to receive the givens of reality, to attend to the reality of sex rather than try to manufacture it. Only that gives each of us a way out of the claustrophobic closet of My Little Universe into the wide sunlit realm of reality.

CHAPTER FOUR

Bobbi and Mike's Story

Bobbi and Mike have traveled both the way of egoism and the way of gratitude.

Bobbi is an outgoing, funny, and enthusiastic woman who works as a youth minister in her parish. She laughs easily and often at her own expense. Her husband, Mike, is more reserved, supplying ballast to the family and tempering Bobbi's inclinations to sudden decisions. During their marriage preparation, they took a Natural Family Planning (NFP) class, which taught them how to avoid pregnancy by abstaining during the woman's fertile times. For the first five or so years of their marriage, they had some wildly haphazard and comedic recourse to the instruction they had received, and a girl, twin boys, and a girl were given to them by the Father in a graciousness that went beyond their planning. With the last pregnancy, they started to panic. "Whoa," Bobbi remembers feeling, "we just cannot have any more kids!"

At that point, pregnant with their fourth child, they were standing outside of church talking to a parish priest. He told them, "You should really think about how to avoid getting pregnant again," reassuring them that whatever happened in their bedroom was between them and God. After all, Bobbi had to be a good wife and mother. With this encouragement, Bobbi and Mike began using condoms.

But it was not as carefree as it was supposed to be. "Even when I was contracepting, I was thinking, did that really work?" Bobbi recollected. "Fear was still involved, because birth control can fail. We were not paying attention to my fertility at that point, and we had no idea where we were in my cycle. We could have been having sex on the most fertile day of the month!"

At this stage in their lives, a seemingly innocuous decision would wind up changing their lives: Bobbi took a class on the *Catechism of the Catholic Church*. In that class she had to face up to the truth that she was not living the way God designed. "Finally, someone challenged us to ask ourselves, 'Why do you think you know better than God?'" Bobbi reported. "Here I was telling teenagers every single day to take God's plan for their lives seriously, and now I wasn't doing it. It was humbling."

In particular, other students in the class lovingly pushed Bobbi to face up to the real motives behind the choice to contracept. "What are you so afraid of?" they asked her. "We talked about it," Bobbi said, "and it really was fear. What if a future baby has problems? What if I can't do it? It all came down to fear of not being in charge. I didn't even know I was so afraid." In that moment, Bobbi decided to let go and let God take over. In class, Bobbi choked up. "I get it," she said, near tears. "It's about trust. It's about trusting God." She went home and told Mike, "I can't contracept anymore."

Mike's reaction? "I hate that class."

But Mike grudgingly agreed to go back to regulating fertility in a non-contraceptive way. At first, Bobbi and Mike used a rough (and extreme) version of the calendar (or rhythm) method. Laughing, Bobbi relates, "Five days after my period and until about day twenty-six, we basically said, 'I'm not coming near you.'" In other words, they felt as though avoiding pregnancy was still of primary importance. But slowly the method began to work on them. "We went from there to 'God, if you want us to be more open to life, you have to change our hearts,'" Bobbi said. "Then to 'if it happens, it happens.' Finally, about nine months later, I said, 'Should we *try* to have a baby?' We went to the drugstore on our date night to get a basal thermometer [in order to practice NFP properly], and we learned we were already pregnant! We were actually relieved. We didn't want having a baby to be a science project: 'I'm fertile right now, honey; you'd better come home!'"

Bobbi is characteristically effusive about how much better their lives are without contraception. "That whole experience of letting go of fear has really changed a lot of other things. We always ask what God's plan is now, and his plan is always so much better. Whether or not we like it, he knows us better than we know ourselves. The fear is just gone. Sometimes it is a little scary, but giving up control is very freeing. A person who can't invite God into an intimate relationship shouldn't be in that relationship. We did not invite God to be involved in our decision to contracept, but we clearly involved him in our decision not to contracept." Then, thinking about her fifth child, she laughs, "We look at this baby every day, and he is clearly sent by God. He has this aura about him, as though he is saying, 'See, God knew better than you did.'"

Mike has also grown through the practice of NFP. Abstaining from sex can be harder for a man. "Not to sound obnoxious, but just going by natural desires, I want what I want when I want it. To have to think about it when I just want to do it can be hard. Sometimes we have to do the right thing even when we don't like it."

The experience has helped him grow in surprising ways. "I have a newfound and deeper respect for Bobbi's understanding of things," he reports. "I can understand her point of view better, even when I don't always like that point of view. I want to do what is right and I've learned to respect what is right, but I don't have to understand it perfectly. But I do it, and I love it, because it is the truth."

Bobbi adds, "The best thing about NFP is that every single month we have to talk about what is most important in life now. With contraception, we didn't have to talk about our budget, whether we could afford another kid, whether I can take time off from work. With NFP, we have to ask: 'Is sex so important at this very moment that we will change our family, or will we do something else to express our love?'"

By contrast, Bobbi and Mike reflected on the sad situation of Mike's brother, who went through a messy divorce recently. Bobbi observes, "I have never met faithful Catholic people really following God's plan who are divorced. When people who are married allow God in them and between them and around them, it usually doesn't end tragically in divorce. We have always been best of friends, but since our conversion away from contraception, I am so much more deeply in love with Mike because I am in love with all of him, even his fertility."

CHAPTER FIVE

God Wants You to Be Happy

The story of Bobbi and Mike reminds us that living in accord with reality is not easy. But it is the better way, because living in an illusion can never satisfy us. We are made for knowing the truth and loving in accord with it. If we treat reality as an oppressive force rather than our best friend, we cannot live fully human lives, because we are built for truth. That's why we have minds and ask questions and why *true* love is always to be found only in the truth.

Human biology has certain definite contours, a certain reality. As animals that can think and love, we are spiritual as well as sexual beings. Our reproductive systems have an anatomical structure and complicated physiological mechanisms designed for the purpose of reproduction. Rather than being passively subject to sexual urges, however, we are the only animals able to understand what sex is about and able to freely choose to act or not to act. That is, freedom is meant to be used to love.

Of course, many of the more complex species feature incipient rational behaviors. But *Homo sapiens* are the only animals who look into the starry heavens and ask *why*? They are the only ones who gaze in wonder at their beloved and ask *why do you exist*? They are the only ones to go through existential dramas and midlife crises. A dog can feel deep canine loss when an affectionate master departs. But the dog does not ask what the meaning of life is, because his horizon does not include *meaning*. Only the rational animal can ask about *meaning*.

As a result, we have an infinitely wider possible range of experience than a dog has. A creature who can ask about meaning can experience the shattering belief that meaning is absent or the joyous affirmation that it exists. Only the rational human person, in other words, is capable of despair and joy. Both despair and joy are directly tied to how we answer the question about meaning.

Meaning is an interesting word. The popes use it to signify a person's true understanding of the world. When I attend to reality, address questions to it, and come to some verified understanding of it, my mind is grasping real meaning. If I believe the world is meaningless, I suspect that the heart of the world is darkness—at best a random process—and that asking and answering questions is a fruitless endeavor. In contrast, the one who is convinced that reality has meaning lives in a different space. His world is shot through with light and intelligibility.

What does all this have to do with sex and contraception? When the Church insists that we *pay attention to reality*—and reality in its givenness, not its parody found in my rationalizations—we can only respond seriously if we have made a decision in favor of *meaning*. If reality is something that has meaning, then it is worth querying. Then our attitude becomes one of humility: What do I have to learn about this reality? It is not that of the egoist: How can I manipulate reality in order to have the experiences I want to have?

This also means a countercultural stance concerning the meaningfulness of sex. Despite the high esteem in which the wider culture supposedly holds sex, the dominant attitude about it is actually one of profound unseriousness. Sex means whatever we want it to mean. It has no basic reality in itself. Sex is the white screen on which we project our hopes, identities, assumptions, and whatever else we want. It is a mirror, not a painting.

Countering this, as we have seen, the Church points out that sex has its own meaning that is not reducible to what I would like sex to be. In fact, it has two meanings: babies and bonding. For a person made to feed on truth and to express this truth in loving well, genuine happiness can be found only in embracing the twofold meaning of sex, even if it is difficult.

Happiness is a hard word to understand rightly. It is easy to think of happiness as the accumulation of as many pleasures as possible. But if we understand that we are rational animals, we will see that true human flourishing must engage those higher faculties of knowing and loving, or else it is not the maximal experience that humans are capable of having. Remember, unlike Fido, we are capable not only of pleasure and pain, but also of joy and despair. A person should aim at joy and not stop short at mere pleasure.

Many people are startled to hear that the Church (and, thus, God) is rooting for our happiness. One of the loudest complaints against Christianity is that it is a killjoy. In fact, God is pro-joy. Our loving Father wants nothing else for us than our enduring happiness, so much so that he won't let us settle for pale substitutes.

The happiness our loving Father has in mind for *you* in particular has a name: your *vocation*. This vocation is God the Father's loving plan for your life. It is not a plan that contravenes the given patterns of the world. Rather, it is a plan that depends on those patterns. Accepting the reality of sex is one crucial step in carrying out the much larger responsibility that each of us has, to accept the reality of the Father's plan in our unique lives. Each of us must ask: Can I trust the Giver of reality?

Chapter Six

Susan and Ed's Story

Unlike Bobbi and Mike, Susan and Ed never used contraception. But like them, they had to learn—concretely, for themselves—that God's way is the best way. That process of realization strengthened their marriage beyond their finest dreams.

Susan comes from a large family, one of eight children. She and Ed have been married now for over twenty-five years. At the beginning of their marriage, Ed didn't want Susan to suffer the side effects of the Pill. Susan knew of Natural Family Planning from her sisters. "I never heard about NFP in church, ever," Susan said. "We took a class in it before we got married. Some would say I flunked because I got pregnant on my honeymoon." This was not their plan. Their plan was for Ed to get his MBA while Susan worked. "We were going to get the nice house in the suburbs," Ed recalled. "We thought it was terrible, horrible, that we got pregnant. But now I realize that it was probably the best thing that ever happened to us." Susan added, "It was as though we thought intercourse didn't cause life. I mean, we knew it, but we didn't know it."

Change happened through prayer. "My selfishness needed to be addressed, and I knew it," Susan said. At five months pregnant, still very sick, she decided to quit her job and prepare for the new baby. "It was a decision, an act of the will," she said. "God removed the obstacles that were in the way of embracing this. Everything became, 'What is God's will for all this?'"

When their second child, a boy, was born, he was very colicky. "It was a really difficult two years," Susan remembered, "and that was when I really learned sacrificial love, going all day with a toddler and all night with a crying baby who never slept through the night— that was when I really learned to pray. I truly believe that all of this was a result of NFP—that I could trust God. The difficulties in parenting helped me to really grow in conversion."

After years of self-sacrificial love in parenting, Susan and Ed had grown so much spiritually that they were able to embrace the other crosses that would come. After their third baby, Ed got laid off, just after they had bought the house of their dreams. "It was a scary time, and we knew Susan couldn't work with a breastfeeding baby," Ed said. He was laid off for a significant amount of time. They had to drop their health insurance because it cost almost as much as their mortgage.

At this point, they asked themselves if they could use birth control. In addition to their financial woes, Susan had health problems that made another pregnancy dangerous. Just as with Bobbi and Mike, a priest told them that they should use contraception. He said that no one would expect them to do otherwise, given their situation.

"I was on the front steps of the church," Susan recalled. "I could have gone either to the drugstore or directly home. I don't know what it was, but my conscience wouldn't allow me to go to the drugstore and get a barrier method." She went home and told Ed, "I think we need more reasons. What has sustained us in our use of NFP isn't working right now and we need to go deeper."

That was pre-Internet, but Susan found a graduate theology student who was willing to do a home study on the topic. A group in Susan and Ed's home studied the creed, Pope Pius XI's letter *Casti Connubii*, Pope Paul VI's *Humanae Vitae*, and Pope John Paul II's *Letter to Families*. "It absolutely changed my life," Susan stated. "Every time we went to the well, we came away with a deeper understanding; it never ran dry. I could not get enough of that class."

The experience taught Susan and Ed that if the sexual aspect of a marriage isn't right, nothing is right. "Just as the grace and order filters out into the family, so too does disorder," Susan said. "NFP taught me to ask: How do we live our life in a way that puts God's will first?" Susan continued to stay home despite considerable financial sacrifice. "We didn't take vacations until later," Ed said. "I'd rather give my kids a sibling than a vacation."

Now that their kids are all grown, Susan and Ed can see the fruit of the selflessness that NFP taught them. Their eldest son is married and using NFP. "My daughter-in-law's family was shocked: 'What is this rhythm thing that she is going to be using?'" they asked, confusing NFP with the older rhythm method. Susan laughed. "Now they are evangelized. Thankfully, God gave us the opportunity to tell the truth in love and patience."

"When I look at my first child, I always say, thanks be to God," Susan said, "because if Ed and I had used birth control, she wouldn't be here." Ed added, "God knew from all eternity that she was meant to be, and thanks be to God we cooperated."

CHAPTER SEVEN

NFP: Not Your Grandmother's Rhythm Method

The couples who have shared their stories are witnesses to what Natural Family Planning (NFP) did for their marriages. If you are thinking, "NFP is just Catholic birth control," well, you are not the only one. Most people think that NFP is an exception to the Church's prohibition of contraception, that it is the only acceptable contraceptive method. But that is incorrect. NFP is not contraception at all; it is a different species altogether. Nor is it the *rhythm method*.

In order to understand what NFP is not, we have to understand what it is. NFP tracks a woman's signs of fertility, which are caused by the changing hormone levels that precede and follow the release of an egg every month. Bill Cosby had a comedy routine that perfectly expressed the reality of cyclical female fertility. The routine went something like this: "The man, he's *constant*. [Slobbering noises.] The woman, she's *fickle*. 'C'mere, c'mere, c'mere! Go'way, go'way, go 'way!'"[1] Cosby was alluding to women's emotional states, but he inadvertently summarized the biological reality as well: as long as a man's reproductive system is healthy, he is always fertile. He is constant. The woman is sometimes fertile, sometimes not. So NFP doesn't bother with the man but pays attention to the woman and her daily signs of fertility. In contrast, *rhythm* relies on a calendar: a woman who menstruates in the first week of the month should avoid sex in the third week of the month. But most women do not have a perfect twenty-eight-day cycle. NFP does not make assumptions about the future but rather judges whether or not a woman is fertile *today*.

When a woman's reproductive system is saying, "c'mere!" the couple trying to avoid pregnancy can avoid the action that leads to pregnancy: sex. But her reproductive system is not always *on*; it is not always fertile. A woman is fertile only when an egg has been released, about five to seven days a month given how long the egg lives and how long sperm can live in the woman's body. Couples highly motivated to avoid pregnancy abstain a little extra on either end of the fertile period just to be doubly sure. For most couples, this means abstaining around seven to twelve days a month. For most of the month, no egg is present to be fertilized, and conception cannot occur.

How do couples know when to abstain? This book cannot go into detail about modern methods of NFP, but more information is easily available. I will just summarize here. Briefly, the hormone levels surrounding the release of the egg every month cause observable physical reactions. There are three basic signs of fertility that NFP methods rely upon: cervical fluid, which provides an environment during the fertile time conducive to the sperm making their way up to the egg; temperature, which remains high for a sustained time when the fertile time is over; and the position of the cervix. The Billings Ovulation and Creighton NFP methods rely on fluid, while the sympto-thermal method taught by the Couple to Couple League uses all three signs. The Marquette method also uses fertility monitors to check hormone levels. It is best if you learn one of these methods from a trained NFP teacher. Search online to learn more, or check your diocesan website to see if an NFP consultant is on staff. The important thing to remember is that NFP really works for avoiding pregnancy. Don't believe it? Look at the statistics: the method-failure rate of the sympto-thermal method of NFP is under 1 percent, comparable to that of the birth-control pill.[2]

If you have been paying attention to my argument about the purpose of sex, you will not be surprised to learn that the woman's "c'mere" and "go'way" stages describe both a woman's fertility as well as her interest in sex. In other words, her most fertile time corresponds to the time of the month when she most wants sex, while her most infertile time is usually when she is least interested. If you are trying to avoid pregnancy, you are probably thinking, "Bummer. That makes life more difficult." But, as we have already seen, sex is a function of your reproductive system, and the goal of that system is to maximize your odds of reproducing. If you want to play the sex-game, you have to play by its rules. If it seems as if the rules are rigged for a particular outcome, they are! Biologically speaking, you win the sex game when you successfully reproduce.

This fact explains what is an otherwise puzzling, if not traumatic, reality: Well-meaning people using birth control often get pregnant. Recall the undergraduate blogger referenced in chapter two who defended her use of contraceptives by stating, "They've allowed me to live my life without the fear of unwanted pregnancies or deadly diseases." Such an assertion seems almost touchingly naïve to anyone who has studied contraceptive failure rates. The Pill's so-called perfect use failure rate is less than 1 percent, but in real life, when real people use it, its failure rate is more like 9 percent. (This is known as the *user-failure* rate in the field of public health.) The condom's *perfect use* failure rate is 2 percent, but in real life, in which condoms break and people put them on wrong, it is, according to some studies, a whopping 18 percent—and that is just the rate at which pregnancies occur.[3] Failure rates when it comes to disease prevention are higher. If a woman really wants to be free of the fear of pregnancy or sexually transmitted infection, she has to do the one thing that guarantees she will not get pregnant or contract an STI: abstain from non-monogamous sexual activity.

But when people like our co-ed blogger are not attuned to the reality that the biological purpose of sex is procreation, they are unequipped to deal with the result when sex accomplishes what it is meant to accomplish, that is, the conception of new human life. Contraception promises something that it cannot deliver: to change the rules of the sex game so that its new goal is no longer procreation but recreation. As Dr. Janet Smith and others have explained, those caught up in contraceptive practice think they have made a bargain: sex with no babies. Like the young blogger, a person using contraception naïvely believes that the reality of sex (for her, at least) is not reproductive. What happens if she *does* reproduce, conceiving a new, unique member of the human species? The birth controller is unprepared for reality. Sex isn't supposed to result in children! But while contraception can hide the reality, at least for a little bit, sex remains oriented to procreation as much as it ever was.

The collision between the inherent reality of sex and the futile denial of that reality explains the otherwise perplexing statistical link between contraceptive usage and abortion. We have all heard the arguments, often from truly well-meaning people, that more contraceptive use would decrease "unwanted pregnancies" and thus abortion. (I used to find this persuasive too.) But it is false: increased contraceptive use is correlated with *increased* abortion. When a person has built a lifestyle upon the shaky "guarantee" of non-procreative sex, he or she is often unable to conceive of a new way of living . . . with a child. Abortion becomes backup birth control. In fact, the Alan Guttmacher Institute (the research arm of pro-abortion Planned Parenthood) reports that 54 percent of women having abortions used contraception *the same month* in which they got pregnant. Only 8 percent of aborting women have *never* used contraception.[4] Contraceptive inexperience is not the issue. Contraception does not prevent abortion. Instead, it makes abortion even more necessary.

In contrast to birth control, NFP recognizes that we are not sorcerers capable of changing the nature of sex; rather, we are receivers of a reality. Instead of fighting to change the meaning of sex, NFP works within that meaning. People using NFP are better equipped to handle the occasional surprise of an unexpected pregnancy, because the whole method depends on the scientific fact that sex is designed to be procreative. NFP prepares its users to welcome life.

CHAPTER EIGHT

NFP: Why Living in Reality Makes Us Happier

A Catholic who has a big family and eschews con-traception has likely had the following experience: Someone dismisses NFP by saying, "But that method doesn't work; look how many kids you have." In response, I like to say, "Define 'work.'" If I had wanted to, in theory, I could have foregone the children I do have by using NFP to avoid pregnancy. But NFP has *worked* on me at a much deeper level.

I grew up with two siblings, one of whom was a late addition. For most of my childhood, I was the girl half of a two-child family. Almost all of my friends' families, headed mostly by professors, were two-child families. The Mormons across the street with four girls were just plain exotic.

My sense of reality began to change when I started researching the twentieth-century eugenics movement and its contraceptive advocacy, a story summarized in the next chapter. Thinkers as irreligious as feminist Germaine Greer gave me a new way to think about motherhood and children. Maybe it was not healthy for women to view their bodies, especially their reproductive systems, with fear and loathing. I also met more young families in which children were being cared for by stay-at-home or work-at-home moms. Then, our loving heavenly Father gave us the gift of our first child.

This gift was the direct result of the flexibility and pedagogy that NFP provides. While I was doing my doctoral coursework, we had a serious reason to avoid pregnancy, and we practiced NFP carefully. But once that reason became less serious, we reassessed our situation and began to *cheat* a little on the margins of my fertility window. This ability to reconsider one's reproductive plans is a great benefit of the method. NFP enables a couple to avoid sexual autopilot. The Pill or, even worse, the IUD or sterilization facilitates oblivion: the user never has to ask the important questions about what God wills for her fertility right then. In contrast, as Bobbi's story shows, NFP-practicing couples tend to address these questions every month, usually right around the fertile time!

My bigger point is that NFP *worked* in a way that statistics can't easily measure. NFP worked on *me* by making me more open to life—more open to the reality of sex itself as procreative. NFP enabled me to welcome the beautiful gifts that are my children, because it made sex not all about me or even about us, but also about children and the future of our love. My fertility is not an annoyance to be controlled but rather a means for God the Father's plan of loving goodness to work itself out in my life.

The communication that NFP facilitates and the growth that it encourages explain why NFP-practicing couples have such a low incidence of divorce—around 2 to 4 percent—while the divorce rate for contracepting couples hovers around 45 percent.[1] NFP fosters happiness in marriage because it promotes human maturity. A person who is willing to welcome children has to be less self-involved and more generous than someone who sets definite limits to accepting children: I'll be this generous, but no more. As numerous studies of marital happiness have shown, generous and selfless people are easier to live with than stingy and selfish people. (Who knew?)

The fact that NFP has positive effects on people, in contrast to contraception, evinces the truth that using NFP is an altogether different reality from contracepting. We find this tough to understand. We are so used to living like egoists instead of grateful receivers that we cannot grasp that actions have a reality that transcends the meaning we want to impose on them. Remember the treatment of meaning in chapter five: meaning is a fruit of the encounter of an attentive and questioning person with the reality of the world. If we do not thoughtfully encounter reality, we cannot understand the world truly. Meaning eludes us.

For the egoist, reality is always constructed, not ever a thing received. All that matters is what happens between our ears. The egoist accordingly finds it hard to see a difference between the person who contracepts and the person who uses NFP to avoid pregnancy, because what happens between the ears—the intention—is the same: both wish to avoid pregnancy. The action must be the same, right?

The grateful person who attentively considers the fabric of the real, however, recognizes that another reality lies beyond what a person simply intends to accomplish with an action. There is the *action itself*. What is the person actually *doing*? Suppose my intention is to nourish myself. I could carry out that intention by making a big salad or by eating sand and seawater. The actions are not equivalent: one promotes my flourishing, the other frustrates it. Or suppose my intention is to get a promotion at work. I could do that by working hard at my job or by destroying a rival coworker through slander. Are the actions the same just because the intention is the same? Of course not, because a person can have a good goal and do either something good or something wrong in order to achieve that goal.

So it is with contraception and NFP. I can have the good goal of avoiding pregnancy at this time for non-frivolous reasons (my intention). Choosing to achieve that goal through abstaining from sex when I am fertile is a much different thing than deliberately trying to make sex non-reproductive. *What* is the contracepting couple doing? Taking a pill or using a barrier to deliberately sterilize their sex act. *What* is an NFP couple doing? Abstaining. The intention might be the same, but there is a big difference between abstaining from sex when one is fertile, and engaging in sterilized sex. Abstaining from sex is not morally problematic; as Christopher West likes to say, we are probably all doing it right now! God does not demand that we engage in sex only when the woman is fertile. If so, he would not make the woman infertile for most of her cycle. NFP honors the reality of the elegant cycling of the fertile female body. Contraception attempts to eliminate the fertility.

Janet Smith counsels people who do not see the difference between NFP and contraception to try NFP. If the methods are the same, you won't notice a difference! But of course the reason we run from NFP is that it really is different, in profound ways, from contraception. Abstinence makes NFP different from contraception. Abstinence also makes NFP good for us, because temporarily sacrificing our desires for a common good makes us selfless and generous people. In other words, it makes us happy. (NFP also differs from contraception in another countercultural way, by channeling sexual desire to make it revolve around the realities of the female body.)

NFP respects the reality of sex and of the female body; it plays by the rules of the sex game. In contrast, birth control tries to change the reality of sex. The first promotes living as grateful receivers of the good and beautiful reality of sex, while the second facilitates living as sexual egoists. No wonder the effects of NFP are so much better. The next three chapters will explore in more depth the adverse effects of contraception on individuals and on society, that is, what happens when just about everyone tries to live out of egoism rather than out of grateful wonder for reality.

CHAPTER NINE

Popes as Prophets

The previous chapters have laid the groundwork for an adequate understanding of our contemporary scene. If contraception encourages people to be egoists, in denial of the realities of sexuality, and if a whole society embraces birth control, then the true contours of sex recede in public consciousness. It is replaced by fantasy: by whatever I want sex to mean.[1] Sex becomes relentlessly me-focused. Sex with someone who thinks sex is mostly about *me* is a lot different from sex with someone who thinks sex is about procreation and faithful love. Which one would you prefer?

I do not mean to say that everyone using contraception is a seething mass of selfish desires, manipulating partners with malicious deliberation. I am not saying that every time someone uses birth control, she is consciously thinking only about herself. What I am saying is that the acceptance of contraception means the acceptance of a certain attitude about sex that places personal and socially conditioned desires ahead of the reality of sex itself as procreative and unitive. It is simply the case that anyone who uses contraception believes that sex need not be reproductive. It does not mean that this person has thought much about it. Indeed, the world is filled with thoughtless sex.

What I do mean to say is that the contraceptive attitude—even if unthinkingly embraced—still harms decent people. The objectively built-in me-centeredness of contraception, even when it is not consciously embraced, eats away at relationships like an acid. Foreseeing this, Pope Paul VI wrote that "husbands who become accustomed to contraceptive practices will lose respect for their wives. They may come to . . . use their wives as instruments for serving their own desires."[2] The pope's language of "husband" and "wife" is already quaint. The breakdown of marriage and the dramatic increase in extramarital sexuality are in fact other effects prophesied by the pope, who called attention to "how easy it [would] be to justify behavior leading to marital infidelity or to a gradual weakening in the discipline of morality."[3] He was especially concerned with how this lax morality would affect the young, noting, "It is wrong to make it easy for them to violate this [moral] law."[4] Lastly, he argued, governments would find it easy to take the step of mandating contraception, for if it is good for women and good for the world, why should something so good be optional? The population-control programs in places like China are blatant examples of the exercise of this dangerous power. Let's not forget, however, the federal government of the United States has made its own attempts to force everyone to pay for contraception, sterilization, and abortion-inducing drugs on the grounds that they are a necessary part of providing for women's so-called health.

The words of *Humanae Vitae* were already countercultural in 1968. Many people have the sense that the Catholic Church is the lone Christian opponent to birth control. In fact, every Christian denomination, including Protestant ones, condemned contraception until 1930, when the Anglican Communion approved its use in limited cases by married couples. This decision opened the floodgates, and all major Protestant denominations followed suit.

Most people assume that Christians have made such determinations based on narrow considerations of sexual morality. That assumption, however, is historically uninformed. It is no accident that the Anglicans came out in favor of birth control in 1930. The 1920s and 1930s were in many ways the high-water mark of the organized eugenics movement, which by that point had mostly embraced birth control as the means to eugenic control in the developed world and abroad. Eugenics is an ideology that divides the world into the *fit*—supposedly those with good genes and traits—and the *unfit*—supposedly those with undesirable characteristics. Eugenicists believe that human problems are passed on through heredity, and want to eliminate social problems by eliminating the people who have those problems.

By the 1920s, most eugenicists had embraced birth control and sterilization as the means to ensure that the *unfit* would not pass on their defective characteristics through reproduction. In the 1970s, abortion was added to the arsenal. Frederick Osborn, the leading American eugenicist from the 1920s until the 1970s, stated forthrightly in 1973 that "birth control and abortion are proving to be great eugenic advances of our time."[5]

By 1930, elite opinion—expressed by the media, college professors, legislators, and so forth—was overwhelmingly pro-eugenic, and any discussion of contraception was undertaken within this eugenic context.

The American Margaret Sanger (1879–1966) spearheaded the movement to promote eugenics via birth control. In 1916 she founded what would come to be called the Planned Parenthood Federation of America (PPFA). Sanger wrote that birth control was "nothing more or less than the facilitation of the process of weeding out the unfit."[6] (In America and abroad, the only organized opposition to her vision was mustered by . . . the Catholic Church.) In 1927 the Supreme Court made its 8–1 *Buck v. Bell* decision, which allowed states to sterilize citizens without their consent and sometimes even without their knowledge. It is estimated that over 67,000 Americans were sterilized under these state laws between 1927 and the 1960s.[7] *Buck v. Bell* was never overturned.

By the 1960s, eugenics was discredited in name but not as an idea. Already in the 1920s, savvy eugenicists such as Sanger were orchestrating a transition from eugenics to population control. While her plan was not widely understood by the public, historians of eugenics know that the eugenics movement and the population-control movement were one and the same. The same activists and organizations constituted both movements. Eugenics sought "quality, not quantity," as one popular slogan put it: eugenic quality, not population quantity. Population control is eugenics with a passport.

Thus, when population control became a dominant public concern in the 1960s, making contraception even more acceptable, eugenics expanded instead of dying away. Concerns about overpopulation, often greased by foundation money, seeped into the thinking of progressive theologians, who drank in eugenics with the potion of pro-contraception ideology. Often-unstated assumptions about the dignity of people of color in the developing world, as well as poor people here, undergirded the demands for contraceptive-enabled population control. People need only read the bestselling *The Population Bomb* (1968) by Paul Ehrlich to acquaint themselves with the rising distaste for the reproduction of nonwhites.

> I came to understand the population explosion emotionally one stinking hot night in Delhi . . . . People eating, people washing, people sleeping, people visiting, arguing, and screaming. People thrusting their hands through the taxi window, begging. People herding animals. People, people, people, people.[8]

Ehrlich had predicted demographically driven mass starvation, but almost immediately after *The Population Bomb* was published, his thesis utterly collapsed. The agricultural innovations constituting Norman Borlaug's Green Revolution had come to fruition. People don't starve because there isn't enough food. People starve because of dysfunctional and corrupt states and because of trade policies that harm developing nations. Given human enterprise and creative ingenuity, the world can support far more than the over seven billion currently alive.

So, far from being a rational concern, overpopulation is the very opposite of what should worry us: overwhelming demographic evidence has mounted that the world is facing a severe depopulation crisis. Stephen Mosher's Population Research Institute has done good work gathering and explaining this data, and I encourage the reader to check it out for more information.[9]

In the 1960s, however, it was not data but ideology that drove the public discussion. An anti-humanist environmentalist ideology looked upon people, especially the poor here and abroad, as problems to be eliminated. Elite opinion was, and indeed still is, avidly in favor of population control—just as it was pro-eugenics in the 1920s and 1930s.

Nevertheless, a quiet tide has been rising against elite control, a countercultural resistance to the social script that says that contraception is to be accepted without critical thinking. Despite the fact that a majority of

Catholics use birth control, more acceptance of Church teaching exists now than at any point since *Humanae Vitae*. Why is the tide starting to turn? The ultimate reason is, of course, the Holy Spirit. And one of the great instruments of the Spirit in this revitalization of sexual authenticity was Pope John Paul II, who provided a joyful witness to the entire truth of the Gospel. He gave us an invaluable gift in his theology of the body, which provided a new lens for understanding *Humanae Vitae* and the Church's teaching on contraception. This book cannot comment on the theology of the body in detail, but the insights provided by John Paul II's theology permeate these pages.

I will mention only one particular theme. Pope Paul VI notes that the key to moral family planning is the self-mastery of free moral agents, "the habit of complete mastery of themselves and their desires."[10] John Paul II fleshes this out in the theology of the body by emphasizing the importance of conversion of the heart, a conversion that enables self-mastery. As the next chapter will explore, both popes are setting up *self-control* as the alternative to *birth control*.

CHAPTER TEN

If Birth Control Is the Solution, What's the Problem?

In order to understand what the popes teach about self-mastery, we have to understand better Margaret Sanger's proposal that contraception is the great solution to social problems. Our society embraces Sanger's worldview without a second thought. It is always helpful to step back and be critically minded. If birth control is the solution, what is the problem?

The problem must be biological; the problem must be fertility. In particular, Sanger insisted, the problem is *female* fertility. Without contraception, women cannot be liberated. If contraception is necessary to bring about female liberation, then what degrades women is . . . female fertility. *Women are oppressed by their own bodies*. Almost all of us believe this. Most of us have not actually thought this through explicitly; rather, it is the air we breathe, the thin aerosol of socially dominant propaganda. It is an unspoken subtext of virtually every movie, TV show, and popular novel. But what does this proposition really say about women?

At the very least, it says that women, especially their bodies, are innately defective. According to the social script by which most Westerners live their lives, female fertility is not a gift to be understood and respected. This is in profound contrast to Natural Family Planning, which encourages such respect through its intelligent awareness of the rhythms of a woman's body (the way of gratitude). Sanger's contraceptive ideology views female fertility as a problem to be eliminated through technology. This involves a drive to manipulate living systems without regard for their reality: this is what egoism looks like when it uses technology to treat life like a designer commodity. The egoistic approach to female fertility fosters discomfort toward the female body, as if it were a problem requiring a technological fix.

The Majority Report of the papal commission whose work preceded the promulgation of *Humanae*

Vitae echoes this attitude when it states that there exists a "duty of man to humanize and to bring to greater perfection for the life of man what is given in nature."[1] (Remember, the commission was considering the question of hormonal contraception for women.) What odd language this is: as though the female body is not already human but somehow requires "humanizing" and "perfecting" via contraception first. And that is not the only example; the Majority Report is shot through with the language of sexual egoism.

In contrast, the popes advocate an intelligent gratefulness toward the body and sex. The body is already good, created by our wise and loving Father; unless diseased or injured, it does not require a technological fix. If we are receptive to the wisely designed gifts that the body and sexuality are, then we will not be tempted to obliterate their reality and meaning by technology.

"Sounds like the Church is against technology," you might protest. "We use technology to manipulate the body all the time, even to the point of neutralizing natural bodily functions. Pain killers disrupt the body's natural pain signaling. What about eyeglasses and artificial limbs?"

It must be understood: the difficulty with contraception is *not* the use of technology as such. Rather, the problem is the misuse of technology. The problem is an uncritical use of technology for egoistic agendas, failing to pay attention to basic features of reality because all the relevant questions are not being asked.

Technology is not the problem. God in fact endowed us with creative intelligence so that we might work in accord with the natures he created: to relieve suffering and to raise the great monuments of civilized life. But in the case of hormonal contraception, technology is being directed against female fertility as if it were a disease, an enemy to be quelled, like suppressing fire. But though female fertility may be threatening to us, female fertility is not disordered in itself.

Some artificial devices, such as eyeglasses, help a bodily organ to function properly. But contraception does not fix a malfunction. A healthy female reproductive system is fertile between menarche and menopause. Contraception actually aims to render a healthy bodily system unable to achieve its goal. Contraception is not like wearing eyeglasses. It is more like amputating a healthy limb. And it is not like using pain killers, because once pain alerts us to a danger, it has served its purpose. Preventing unnecessary pain is a great good even in light of the purpose of pain itself, which simply serves physical integrity. In contrast, preventing reproduction as one engages in a reproductive act (that is, sex) frustrates the whole purpose of a reproductive system.

As Pope Paul VI notes, we cannot do something wrong in order to achieve something good; the end does not justify the means. If we want to achieve the goal of a healthy family life (our intention), we have to do something good (such as NFP) to get there.

NFP is good not because it is somehow non-technological. In fact, it depends on the scientific advances that allowed us to come to understand ovulation and the intricacy of the female reproductive system. The *natural* in Natural Family Planning may be misleading because it might give the inaccurate impression that its moral value lies in its being untouched by technology, which is simply not the case. NFP is good because it depends on our being attentive to the reality of sex and working with that reality rather than trying to obliterate it. NFP doesn't make the mistake of treating female fertility as if it were a disease. And it doesn't try to short-circuit the hard human work of becoming a happy person through a technological fix. No technology can make us happy. The only way to be really happy is to be virtuous. That is, the only way to happiness is by performing good actions and thereby becoming selfless, generous, and loving—the kind of person we all find attractive.

That is, NFP promotes *self-control*, not *birth control*. *Birth* control says that the body is defective and must be fixed; the problem is the body. *Self*-control, instead, says that the problem is the heart, which often is torn by desires running contrary to the demands of real love, the demands of self-sacrifice. If the problem is the heart and not the body, the solution is not to *fix* the body technologically but rather to *convert* the heart. NFP trains my desires, my heart, to be in accord with the reality of sex as procreative and unitive. It trains me to want what is good and what will (therefore) make me truly happy. Contraception simply tries to change sex, leaving my heart untouched. No wonder it solves nothing in the end, as a cursory glance at our society indicates.

CHAPTER ELEVEN

Life in Contraception Land

If the problem is selfishness in the human heart and not the design of the human body, then any authentic solution must address the heart.

This approach clarifies what to the general culture are inexplicable Catholic positions. Let's take the prohibition on using condoms to deal with the AIDS crisis in Africa. We have to remember, first, that even at the technological level, the condom "solution" does not work—remember user and method failure? Recall that the failure rate of condoms in preventing pregnancy in normal use is an unimpressive 18 percent. But of course a condom might leak with no pregnancy resulting, since a woman is fertile less than half the time anyway.

Unlike pregnancy, though, disease can occur anytime user or method failure occurs: so, we're talking about *at least* a nearly one-in-five chance of getting a potentially deadly disease with a condom. Is this really the sound basis of a public-health program? This truth explains why HIV-infection rates in Africa remain high despite its being flooded with condoms.

By the way, many other diseases are transmitted not by secretions but by skin-to-skin contact with lesions—which could be in an area not covered by a condom. Such diseases include genital herpes, chancroid, syphilis, and HPV. Unless the sexual partners are completely wrapped in latex—which is not very sexy— a barrier approach can't prevent all diseases, even when the condoms are in perfect condition and used correctly 100 percent of the time. And how often does that happen?

The deeper reason why condoms cannot *solve* the AIDS crisis (if we bracket the issue of possible medical transmission) is that the problem of sexually transmitted infection is not a bodily problem but a problem of the heart. The only sure-fire way to avoid STIs is fidelity to a single sexual partner who is also faithful. One does not catch an STI except through sex with multiple sexual partners or with a single partner who has had other partners. Condoms are likely to *facilitate* the spread of HIV, because they encourage complacency. A person is given the false assurance that a lifestyle of multiple sexual partners can be disease-free. Unlike, say, the flu, an STI is a lifestyle disease. A person who avoids the lifestyle will not get an STI. But in order to avoid the lifestyle, a person needs to have his or her heart touched. That is why the only successful AIDS-prevention programs targeting the sexual behaviors of the general public have been those that emphasize being faithful to one partner (such as the program promoted in Uganda in the 1990s).[1]

The most dreaded sexually-transmitted condition in America, though, seems not to be a disease but pregnancy. If we cared more about preventing disease rather than pregnancy, NFP's superiority would be manifest. But as the means for most couples to avoid pregnancy, NFP doesn't seem generally attractive. It is often objected that NFP requires too much maturity and commitment from people. But do we need to have contraception in order to enable teens to have one-night stands? Or to enable married couples to avoid talking with each other about fertility, finances, and the future? Think what this means: We are willing to settle for dysfunctional, selfish relationships rather than making clear the kind of commitment and solicitude, the true love, that should be the context of sexual activity.

Contraception has become the societal enabler of sexual immaturity and abuse. Is that really an argument in its favor?

In any case, birth control has done a terrible job of preventing pregnancy among uncommitted or immature partners. Adolescents are particularly bad users of birth control. The Centers for Disease Control reports that "virtually all sexually experienced teenagers have used some method of contraception."[2] We have achieved nearly complete contraceptive saturation among adolescents, and they are still getting pregnant and contracting STIs. The results are not much better among adults; non-marital births are becoming the norm, with all the problems that come with that. A *majority*—more than half—of the babies born to women under 30 are born into single-parent households, and 72 percent of black children do not have both parents at home. Only college-educated women are likely to get married before having children. "Marriage has become a luxury good," said Frank Furstenberg, a sociologist at the University of Pennsylvania.[3]

Why should we care? Well, children born into single-parent (usually single-mother) families are much more likely to be impoverished, to have poor psychological and emotional development, and to do worse in school.[4] These effects last into young adulthood, when these children are less likely to be in school or to have a job. The poverty that a single mother is likely to face impacts her as well, cutting off her opportunities for educational development. That is not to say that many single mothers do not do heroic and near-miraculous jobs raising their children. My husband was raised by his widowed mother and still escaped the poor outcomes that he was statistically likely to suffer. Statistics are not destiny. But they do show that kids who beat the odds have done just that—escaped a fate that most of their peers will suffer.

The takeaway point is that the availability of contraception has not eliminated the possibility of single motherhood. Rather, contraception has *facilitated* it. Birth control has broken down society's acceptance of sex as innately reproductive and thus as something to be reserved for the context in which children are best raised, namely marriage. Contraception has yanked sex out of marriage by trying to rewrite the rules of sex and make it about recreation, not procreation and union. If a couple is not mature and committed enough for children, no problem: they can still have sex—and no kids! But, as we have seen, pregnancy happens anyway, and in fact (as I will show) many young women are not fully committed to avoiding pregnancy, regardless of their marital status. The contraceptive bargain—no more pregnancy in non-ideal situations!— turns out to be a naïve illusion.

Take Amber Strader, 27, who has had two children out of wedlock with two different men. The first boyfriend was so immature she would never consider marrying him. "It was like living with another kid," she said.[5] With her second boyfriend, she was willing to marry, but he was not. How did she get pregnant the second time? Her contraception failed. Birth control did not prevent these births. It just chipped away at the social taboo against having sex outside of marriage, in this case with a man so immature that she had to buy his cigarettes for him. Why would a woman consider having sex with someone like that? It is only possible when sex no longer means an implicit recognition that children might result. It is only possible in a contraceptive world, which tries to pretend sex is about recreation, not procreation.

Amber's situation results in part because contraception cannot eliminate the desire for children, especially on the part of women. When Kathryn Edin and Maria Kefalas described the interviews they had with single mothers they summarized the data as follows: "While the poor women we interviewed saw marriage as a luxury, something they aspired to but feared they might never achieve, they judged children to be a necessity, an absolutely essential part of a young woman's life, the chief source of identity and meaning."[6]

What contraception has done to impact the lives of these women has largely occurred prior to their own sexual activity: it has broken down the social script built on recognition of sex as procreative, with its proper context in marriage. These women still want children (contraception hasn't changed that), but marriage has become a distant reality, one they can't seem to achieve. Birth control has enabled men to get sexual gratification without the hassle of lifelong commitment. What is the result? No one is being trained to be a good spouse, but everyone is being sexualized. So the women settle for the sex and the children, while wondering if Prince Charming will ever come someday. As we saw with HIV, so too here: rather than eliminating behavior that harms individuals and society (especially women and girls), contraception enables it.

In fact, single moms are right: children are a great good. With single motherhood and teenage pregnancy, the problem is not pregnancy; motherhood is a beautiful thing. The problem is the nonmarital sex, that is, sex without committed love that is the context for the pregnancy. Contraception and abortion have facilitated, even encouraged, risky sexual behavior, which is defined as sex that has a high likelihood to lead to disease, unplanned pregnancy, and/or personal danger.

This effect is seen especially in the young, who are the most vulnerable to the negative impacts of sex outside of loving commitment. Sexually active teens do worse in school, are less likely to attend college or graduate, more likely to be depressed, and more likely to commit suicide. Adolescent sexual activity is a huge public-health problem. One study has found that "the younger a girl is when she begins engaging in sexual activity, the more likely she is to be a risk taker, have poorer judgment, or come to early initiation through a history of sexual abuse that would orient her toward older partners."[7] This only makes sense: just think of all the emotional complications that come with sexual relationships, which distract adolescents from the truly important things on which they should be concentrating (such as studying and developing serious friendships).

These emotional complications have a biological basis. The hormone oxytocin is released during sexual activity. Oxytocin is a bonding hormone: it is also released during pregnancy and breast-feeding, for example, to bond the mother to her baby. Females are particularly impacted by oxytocin during sex. Once again, we see that—despite our intentions or our plans—sex has its own rules. Our very bodies work against some kind of hookup world of baby-free, bonding-free sex. Teenage girls are no exception to the rule, and no amount of contraception is going to protect their *hearts* from experiencing the reality of the bonding aspect of sex.

The bonding that happens in sex can cause plenty of emotional distractions and make break-ups miserable, but it is probably not enough to hold a couple together when things get rough. For long-lasting love and commitment—the kind of love that most people say they want, even if they think it is an unattainable dream—a couple needs sex to be within the context of mature, self-giving, publicly promised love.

So, what about contraception in marriage? Contraception was supposed to make it easier for couples to grow in intimacy and love by enabling more frequent sex without the worry of having too many children. Marriages should have been strengthened. Did it work?

Even a glance at the divorce rate indicates otherwise. In the 1950s and early 1960s, the divorce rate was around 25 percent of all marriages. Beginning around 1968, the rate began a steep upward climb to over 50 percent in 1976, and has hovered at those levels ever since. This climb coincides exactly with the time in which hormonal contraception gained widespread acceptance in American society. Distinguished economist Robert T. Michael has carefully examined the reasons for the sudden rise and leveling-off of the divorce rate. He argues that the contraceptive revolution began to impact America most substantially in 1968 and that, by the late 1970s, the country reached a saturation point: the percentage of people who were likely to use birth control had been reached. The divorce rate tracked alongside the contraception rate. Michael estimated that roughly half of the rise in the divorce rate was due to the new contraceptive technology, since the presence of children decreases the possibility of divorce, while contraception makes marriages less child-centered.[8] When sex's connection to the future and to something beyond me is willfully severed, sex tends to become more selfish. And to repeat the obvious conclusion of modern sociology, selfish people are less likely to have successful relationships than generous people.

This truth is brought home concretely by Dr. Edward N. Peters, a canon lawyer who in his work examined around 1,500 petitions for declarations of nullity (popularly known as annulments). He observed that all but one or two of the couples were using contraception (a percentage close to 100 percent, while the percentage of married couples using contraception in the general public is more like 85 percent). While he acknowledges that cause and effect cannot be directly proven, he asserts, "In my experience, no single factor as directly and as gravely injurious to marriage as taught by [the] Church occurs nearly as frequently in the histories of those who eventually divorce as does contraception."[9] He concludes that, even if birth control does not directly cause divorce, it certainly does nothing to prevent it and in fact encourages the unhealthy attitudes that make divorce more likely.

> Personally, I do not think the decision to use contraception *causes* the decision to divorce. Rather, I think the choice to contracept is the fruit of the same mentality that so often eventually prompts the decision to divorce, especially when contraceptive use predates the wedding. The fundamental self-centeredness (whether morally imputable to the individual or not) of contraception, the grave ignorance about the ends of natural, to say nothing of Christian, marriage which it betrays, the specific attitudes toward children which it evidences, all of these factors are consistent with a predisposition for divorce.[10]

This analysis points out that, in a world plagued by commitment-less sex, divorce, the sex trade, abortion and other violence against children, and less-than-optimal family structures, seeing contraception as the solution means that the social problem has been very narrowly defined: the possibility of disease and pregnancy. (How sad that the two are lumped together with such ease!) We have seen that contraception has a pathetic track record in eliminating these problems. Instead it facilitates a lifestyle that has led, and can only continue to lead in the future, to more disease and crisis pregnancy.

Yet even worse is the very formulation of the problem. If the problems with the sexual revolution are only bodily and technical, then the only solution will be bodily and technical. But it is manifest that the much deeper problems of the current sexual regime are the heartache, narcissism, and nihilism that it breeds. The narrowness involved in reducing what ails us to whatever contraception can supposedly cure is redolent of Margaret Sanger. She narrowed the fight for women's liberation to the right to eliminate one's fertility, scapegoating female fertility as the source of social problems. Sanger's vision still holds sway in our culture, which continues to recognize only one solution to social problems, the contraceptive "solution." It leaves women and girls beaten down, used up, and broken, alone with their Pills. I believe our intellectual complacency has failed women and girls, who deserve better.

We should not forget that this turn of events is quite recent in the history of humanity. It dates, in fact, to the widespread use of contraception, beginning in the 1960s. For millennia the specific contours of sex were recognized, if not always honored: sex is innately reproductive and unitive and hence should be reserved for people ready to accept children in a publicly committed relationship. Of course extramarital sex happened, but it did not happen as often as today, and without the almost total societal acceptance it has now. Societal attitudes changed when, as Pope Paul VI predicted, having sex without children was made easy. Except it is not so easy, as the surge in single-parent families and abortions testify. What changed was not the reproductive nature of sex but our attitudes about it: too many people became sexual egoists rather than people intelligently receptive to the nature of sex. The good news is that attitudes can be changed again, even if it be a steep, uphill battle. We can begin with ourselves and our children.

CHAPTER TWELVE

Responding to Objections to Church Teaching

If you have been reading attentively thus far, you have the tools to answer the objections of Catholics like Daniel Maguire, who was introduced in chapter two. Recall that Maguire claims that Church teaching on contraception arises out of the prejudice that women are evil and that "only reproduction could justify sexual collusion" with them. It is in fact the contraceptive mentality that scapegoats and demonizes the female body, which is seen as a problem requiring the technical solution of birth control. The truth is that our world says too often that only the guaranteed *absence* of reproduction justifies sexual intercourse with women.

That explains the varieties of non-coital sexual activity in currency today, such as the porn lifestyle or what Planned Parenthood promotes as "outercouse," specifically for avoiding the risk of pregnancy. In fact, the Church alone upholds what reason sees: the beautiful design of the female body and of sex.

The Church's actual attitude toward women is expressed in John Paul II's language of the "feminine genius," which embraces female uniqueness, rather than trying to destroy it.[1] Men and women are not simply interchangeable. Science continues to reveal more and more about how men and women are distinct, down to every cell in their bodies. Distinction does not have to mean inequality. The problem of sexism from which women and girls have suffered for so much of human history cannot be solved by pretending that men and women are actually the same thing. It can only be solved by respecting the uniqueness of women— including their fertility, which is an integral part of their bodily existence.

Female dignity can be respected even more when the unique vocation of each woman and girl is understood. Women are not reducible to the kind of sexual pleasure they might bring; they are not mere objects to be enjoyed and discarded, as the contraceptive culture facilitates in the sexual revolution. Each one is a daughter of her loving Father in heaven, who has a particular plan for her. Each plan, each mission, will be irreducibly unique, but each one will involve the generous gift of herself, whether in marriage, religious life, or a form of life in the world shaped by some other kind of public promise to God. (And lest this seem sexist, men also cannot be the persons they are meant to be without the same kinds of self-gift.)

If a woman is called to marriage and is able to have children, the number of children she will receive is also stored in the heart of her loving Father, in the wise and surprising designs of his providence. The Church does not provide a tidy formula by which we can figure out the optimal size of our family. It doesn't say if we have an income of X and our health is Y, the number of children we should have is Z. This intimate calling can only be received, not calculated, and it is received through a loving, mature relationship with one's spouse and a robust prayer life. The Church most certainly does *not* say that a woman must have as many children as she is physically capable of bearing. Procreation is but the first step in the parents' responsibility toward their children. The second, enduring, task is education in the good, preparing children to receive at each moment the grace that will make them saints. Procreation is not an end in itself but serves the ultimate desire of the Father toward each person: to make of that person a saint, uniquely powerful and creative in the Spirit of Jesus Christ.

By contrast, a radically contracted worldview is on display when some people, including many theologians, insist that here-and-now utility is all that matters. They claim that a vague overall openness to life within a whole marriage justifies the occasional or even frequent use of contraception. But even if we grant that it is acceptable to think that the moral value of our actions stems only from adding up how well they serve my current convenience, the argument still does not work. These theologians ignore the harm that the contraceptive attitude does to a marriage, as the previous chapter showed.

At a deeper level, the problem with this way of thinking is that it lumps together good acts with those that are wrong, hoping that the net result will be more good than evil. Do we do this in other areas of the ethical life? Do we figure that, as long we are honest employees the majority of the time, the occasional embezzlement is fine? Or, to take the other meaning of marriage, do we surmise that one or two adulterous affairs do not affect our overall commitment to marital fidelity? Hopefully not, because we should recognize that each and every one of our actions has moral weight, and not just in the aggregate. So, even if a little embezzling would seem to serve the greater good of a financially secure family, the honest businessman refrains from it and finds another way of achieving his good goal. Remember chapter eight: a good intention is not enough; a good kind of *action* is also necessary.

At this point we come back to the issue of why people go to such lengths to insist on contraception over Natural Family Planning. Our culture seems to think that abstaining from sexual activity for just about anyone, at almost any age, and in almost any condition of life, is some kind of unthinkable tragedy. Planned Parenthood style sex education gives the impression that abstinence will make you some kind of weird, repressed misfit. Yet even the most promiscuous of us practice sexual abstinence *sometimes*. Sex is not like breathing: it is okay to take an occasional break from it. Couples practicing NFP take their sex-breaks consecutively. As it happens, contracepting couples do not actually have *more* sex than NFP couples. NFP couples just time their sex differently.

Such periodic abstinence from sex serves a valuable purpose in marriage: it reminds us that our desires are not the last word. Even more, the ability to say no to our desires, even to good and healthy desires, makes us better people who are able to do hard things when necessary and to place the beloved's good before my own. What happens if a spouse becomes ill and cannot have sex? Or has a difficult pregnancy? How much easier it is to abstain during those times, without resentment and without weakening of marital affection, if the couple has some experience of voluntary periodic abstinence. In fact, such occasional abstaining is so helpful to marriage that John Paul II recommends it to *all* married couples, regardless of their wishes concerning pregnancy, as an intrinsic part of a marital spirituality.[2] He proposes this as a way of keeping sex from becoming a mere habit, the scratching of an itch, and as a way of unleashing other "manifestations of affection"[3] that may have fallen away after the first stages of being in love. (Those would be things like the flowers or the specially made dessert that appears in courtship and then sometimes mysteriously disappears after the wedding date.) For couples seeking to avoid pregnancy, the periodic continence built into NFP is especially liberating for women. A couple attuned to the woman's fertile cycles allows its sex life to be structured not by male desire but by the female body.

As we know from other spheres of life (such as eating), occasionally saying "not now" to our desires makes us healthier, more mature people. It makes us selfless. And don't forget what those sociologists say: selfless people are happier and have better relationships.

CHAPTER THIRTEEN

What Should I Do Next?

Perhaps at this point, dear reader, you need a pep talk. You may have considered realities that are new to you. The argument of the book is that it is better to live as grateful recipients of reality than as sexual egoists. Hopefully you found this argument convincing, or at least worth a trial run. Perhaps you were already on board with Catholic teaching but did not understand it as deeply as you wanted to, or else you felt you could not explain it to others. What do you do now? Recall the two powers that human beings have that make them distinct from other animals: knowing and loving. The answer to "what's next?" is to engage both your intellect (knowing) and your will (loving) in the service of the truth.

This book has made a case to your intellect, so you have already been engaging your mind. I will talk more about what your mind can do in a moment. First, let's explore how you can activate your will—your free choices—as a means of helping you to live in accord with the reality of sex as unitive and procreative.

The first step is to give up. By that I do not mean to give *in*, namely, to surrender to desires that are not in tune with reality. Rather I mean to give *up*, that is, to give up control of your life to your loving Father in heaven. As I noted in the first chapter, contraception is often the last holdout for Catholics who assent to Church teaching on just about everything else. The reason is that birth control promises *control* over the most intimate areas of our life, and it therefore promises control of our life as a whole. "I'll listen to you concerning everything else, God," we think, "but I just *know* that I cannot handle any more children, so I need to assert my will in this one area." It is as if we have to tell God what is and is not good for us. We have not yet let go, because we cannot ultimately trust God. We sense he wants to pull us beyond mediocrity, and we fear what that will look like. Giving in to God feels like death.

In fact it is the beginning of life. The happiness that our all-powerful and all-loving Father has in store for us cannot be achieved in us if we allow ourselves to remain cramped and shrunken, busily ruling our little corner of the world. The happiness he has in mind for us is too great to be poured into such an inadequate receptacle. Surrender stretches us to new personal expansiveness. John Paul II speaks of the layers of the personality that are unearthed in those—the saints—who have allowed God to mold them. Can I trust that God the Father will carefully tend me as a master gardener does with a delicate flower, causing my full beauty to blossom, while protecting me from the winds and storms?

"But what if God asks of me something I don't think I can handle?" you might ask. Well, maybe he will, and maybe he won't. I do not know what he has in store for you. But we must be convinced that we will be able to do whatever he calls us to do because he is always there to help us. In fact, we will *only* become truly happy in doing so. This is certain: If we try to thwart God's will in the most intimate areas of life, we are trying to thwart his will for our life. Period. We cannot pick and choose; anything less than complete surrender is no surrender at all. And living without surrender is a sure ticket to unhappiness.

How to do it, then? Simply put, invoke God's power. The first step is more faithful adherence to the

sacraments and, along with that, a growing engage-
ment in prayer. While total surrender is needed, God
meets us where we are and leads us gently closer to
union with him. If you are convinced that surrendering will not be easy for you—and for whom is it
easy?—inform him that he had better enable you to
do it. (At least, that is how I often pray.) A robust
prayer life is necessary, marked by confidence in calling out to the Lord. And such a prayer life grows from
faithful reception of the sacraments. In addition to
the sacrament of Matrimony, two others that must be
mentioned are *Confession* and *the Eucharist*.
Confession is both humbling and revealing—two
things we need very much if we are to be humble
enough to receive grace, and self-aware enough not to
put ourselves in danger of sinning. The grace of
Confession releases us from our burdens and enables
us to start afresh, enveloped by God the Father's
mercy. To be forgiven is one of the deepest needs in
our aching hearts, and in Confession, we hear Jesus
literally tell us, through the priest, that he has forgiven us. The Eucharist then feeds the incipient life of
virtue in us, strengthening us to endure temptation at
least for just one more day. Gradually, virtue will
grow in us, enabling us to do the good with ease, joy,
and promptness, as Saint Thomas Aquinas puts it.

For ultimately virtue, not just abstinence, is our goal. God does not want us to live with perpetual teeth-gritting, saying "no" to bad sex but never saying "yes" to anything. Virtue is saying "yes" to God, so that saying "no" to sin becomes one easy, joyous moment along the way of his will for us. Think of Mother Teresa or Pope John Paul II: the ease with which they said "no" to any temptation to put self-gratification before self-gift was a small moment in their overall "yes" to the greatness of God's will. Saying "no" to egoism is always necessary, but it is not the whole moral life. Our Father wants our "no" to serve a much larger "yes" that is the mission he has chosen for each one of us.

Another way to surrender and say "yes" to God's will is to practice sacrificial *tithing*. I have already observed how money and sex are related. Both are about control of my life and my future. If I am having a hard time surrendering my sexual life to God, it will help if I practice surrender by giving him my financial life. The traditional recommendation for tithing is 10 percent of our income, to be given first to your parish and diocese and then to other worthy charities. Remember that account in which Peter asks about paying the temple tax? Jesus tells him to go fishing, open the mouth of the fish he catches, and use the gold coin he will find therein to pay the tax. This story relates many things, not the least of which is that God has a sense of humor. Another is that money is easy for God. He can invent it out of nothing if he needs to, and we need to trust him with our money. Surrendering our money is good practice for surrendering our lives.

Prayer, the sacraments, and tithing are necessary for us to be able to surrender our lives to God. *Community support and mentorship* are other indispensable means of living in accord with the reality of sex. Seek out like-minded people, especially couples if you are married, or chaste singles if you are single. Find them in your parish, in Catholic online forums, or in home-schooling groups. Imitate their good examples and go to them when you need advice and support. And I will pray for you as well!

These are some strategies for engaging your will. What about your intellect? A first step is *becoming educated*, which hopefully this book has served. The appendix of this book lists other resources for learning more about God's plan for our sexuality. And don't forget the *Catechism of the Catholic Church* (CCC), which is an indispensable resource for learning what the Church teaches about God, creation, the moral life, worship, and prayer. You can find it online or purchase a bound copy.[1] The CCC is such a gift for the layperson!

It empowers you to learn about the faith directly, without having to depend on often unreliable intermediaries such as the media or possibly dissenting theologians. Consider taking a class, either in the classroom or online, to learn more about the riches of the *Catechism*.

The next necessary step is to *spread the truth*. We are first called to evangelize those closest to us. If you have children or grandchildren, help them to understand the reality of sex from the get-go. With younger children, look for informal teaching opportunities to point out that the basic reality of marriage is love and life. Picture books that feature parents with babies or children provide an opportunity to reinforce this: "See how the mommy and daddy love the baby? Their love for their baby and their love for each other go together."

For children old enough to know about sex—and be sure that you are the one introducing the topic for the first time, and not their peers or teachers—emphasize the two meanings of sex: babies and bonding. Help them to see that sexual union is so uniquely powerful in expressing love precisely because it is the kind of act that can give rise to a new life, a life that is the very embodiment of the man and woman's love for each other. Sex belongs in marriage because marriage is the only relationship made for raising children in an atmosphere of true love. Challenge media that present only one side of the story: in reality, would those promiscuous characters be as carefree as they seem? What about disease and heart-break? Better yet, do not let media influences become the parent and teacher of your children. One of the best things my husband and I did was to refuse to get cable TV and video games. This move involved sacrifices for us, the grown-ups, but it has amply paid us back with children who are able to concentrate, think for themselves, and have a healthy sense of love and relationships.

Along those lines, one of the most important things we can do for our children is to *provide an atmosphere* in which the virtues of piety and chastity are possible. The gradual change in my beliefs on contraception was influenced by my studies of Margaret Sanger and eugenics. But it was also an eventual acceptance of a more basic truth: that the Catholic Church was established by Christ and does not err in matters of faith and morals. I did not have to fully understand all her teachings, but I could accept them.

What about reaching those who are not family? First, *understand* where people are coming from. The widespread misconception is that Church teaching on sex only says "no" to our fun. Catholics need to reframe the debate in terms of true happiness (and not just passing pleasure). The *Catechism of the Catholic Church* tells us, "The desire for God is written in the human heart, because man is created by God and for God; and God never ceases to draw man to himself. Only in God will he find the truth and happiness he never stops searching for."[2] This is good news! We must have faith that the person we are evangelizing has deep questions (which might be very deeply buried), questions that only find their answers in Jesus Christ. If we come across as finger-wagging moralists, no one will listen to us. But if we present an alternate path to genuine human happiness, we might be listened to—especially if we have been open to God's grace working in our lives first. As Pope Paul VI reminded us, people today are more willing to listen to witnesses than to teachers, and they will only listen to teachers if they are also witnesses.[3] Once we are credible witnesses, we can use *conversations and social media* to plant seeds. Catholic podcaster Pat Gohn has suggested a "media tithe": give 10 percent of our media use to God. Can we use 10 percent of our social-networking posts to evangelize? These tools, while not without dangers, give us powerful means of reaching people with the Gospel if we use them prayerfully.

Think too about your *parish*. Talk to your pastor about starting a six-week study group on this book or on *Women, Sex, and the Church*, also published by Pauline Books & Media with an online study guide. Make this book and other good resources available. Janet Smith's best-selling talk "Contraception: Why Not?" is available as an inexpensive CD or as a free download. Many people have picked up a copy at the back of their church and had their lives changed by this resource.

Whatever you are able to do, do it with prayer and purpose. It is not our job to change someone's heart; that is for the Holy Spirit. But be convinced that he wants to use you as his instrument. Just ask him how.

CHAPTER FOURTEEN

Secondary Fruitfulness
for the Newly Convinced

The last chapter emphasized the importance of conversion and witness in evangelizing the truth of the life-giving reality of sex. If we are joyful witnesses to living the way of grateful attentiveness rather than the way of egoism, we have a chance of being heard by a hostile world. But what if we have not always lived our own lives in accord with Church teaching? What if you, dear reader, have only become convinced of its truth just now, in reading this book? In this chapter, I would like to pay attention to your situation in particular: the situation of the newly convinced.

A concept from chastity programs for adolescents might be helpful here. Such programs often encourage *secondary virginity*, which is a commitment to begin living chastely again, putting aside the past and accepting the great forgiveness that our heavenly Father wants to lavish on each one of us, no matter our histories. Something similar is relevant to living the way of grateful attentiveness after having wandered on the way of egoism in our sex lives; let us call it *secondary fruitfulness*.

The starting point, once again, is the sacrament of Reconciliation or Confession. It is not the case that God wants to see us beaten down by guilt (the phenomenon of "Catholic guilt" notwithstanding). True, the Church is one of the few voices pointing out that it is necessary to feel guilt when we in fact have failed in the demands of love (and, for us fallen human beings, that is often). The point, however, is that guilt is a means, not an end. Guilt ought to function in a way analogous to that of pleasure in eating or in sex: it is meant to be an impetus for action. In the case of guilt, the action is to ask for forgiveness, ideally in the sacrament of Confession, which Catholics are blessed to have available to them. Guilt is supposed to be a spur, not a perpetual state. If you find you are living in a perpetual state of guilt, God wants to give you a taste of his peace surpassing all understanding, in the great Sacrament of Mercy.

Then what? It is a lot easier to continue a way of living than to turn and set out on a new trajectory. When we have been living contrary to reality, as when using contraception, it is hard to change. A boat chugging along downstream will continue forward by its momentum even if its engine stops. If the boat has to stop midstream and turn around, the process is much more laborious. So it is with us. The Church has traditionally called virtues and vices habits, not to imply they are insignificant tics like nail-biting, but to indicate that we become *habituated* to acting in a certain way. Actions we repeat tend to become second nature. Our character is shaped by our characteristic actions. Remember Saint Thomas Aquinas's definition: a virtuous person acts virtuously with ease, joy, and promptness. For example, it is easy for an honest person in ordinary circumstances not to steal. He has the habit of being honest. In contrast, it is laborious to strike out, as you are doing, on a new path, this path of secondary fruitfulness.

But it won't always be laborious. Walking the way of secondary fruitfulness becomes easier the more one lives it. Beyond the obvious—not using contraception and not engaging in sex outside of marriage—we can take some steps to make it easier. If you aren't married and have been sexually active and contracepting, begin with your sexual habits. Here are some concrete actions to take to make it easier to *live chastely* and therefore to become truly fruitful in love:

❖ Stop cohabitating. It is unrealistic to expect to live chastely in the same domicile as your (former) sexual partner. See some of the tips for married couples (p. 105) to learn how to express love without using sex.

❖ Start discerning marriage. If you have a regular sexual partner, is this someone with whom you should be contemplating marriage? If you know right away that the answer is "no," break it off. If the answer is "maybe," establish a routine of chastity and then begin to discern, with the help of spiritually wise people, what God wants from this relationship.

❖ Be careful with media use. If the computer has been a source of unchastity, especially with porn, how can you find a way to limit its use and to create safeguards for yourself, such as software that blocks porn, for protection in moments of weakness?

❖ Think about people, places, and things. Do your friends make it easier or harder for you to live chastely? Are the environments in which you spend free time conducive to chastity? What do you do when lonely?

❖ Use alcohol responsibly. Nothing makes self-control more difficult than inebriation. Enough said.

What if you are married? Assuming your spouse is on board with secondary fruitfulness, here are some ideas for change:

❖ Dump the barrier methods. Even having them in your house will be a temptation to use them. Besides, do you want your kids to find them?

❖ Get off the Pill. This assumes that there is no underlying medical condition that makes hormonal therapy necessary. If you are treating a medical problem with a medicine that has contraceptive side-effects, you are not contracepting. Treating a medical condition is a different action than deliberately sterilizing the sex act; the former is moral, while the latter is not. That being said, don't be afraid to seek out a Catholic doctor and get a second opinion on hormonal therapy. The Pill has become a go-to medical treatment when it is often not needed. Find a physician who really understands a woman's cycle and is sympathetic to NFP by visiting FertilityCare.org.

❖ Learn NFP as soon as possible. Work with a trained NFP provider if you really want the method to work.

❖ Talk about your fertility plans. Have you made the decision to avoid pregnancy based on outdated considerations? Are economic, physical, or emotional realities you once faced now less pressing? Can you see in what ways the initial decision to contracept was not made in a spirit of receptivity to God's will? Be willing to reassess fertility plans continuously in light of the Father's plan for your family.

❖ Develop habits of asceticism. Learning self-control in other areas will make sexual self-mastery easier. Can I periodically give up caffeine, dessert, taking elevators, or other comforts? How about abstaining from meat on Fridays or fasting on bread and water a day or two a week? How about a media fast (no email, TV, or internet) on Sundays?

❖ Commit to Mass and to prayer time as a couple and family. Being consciously focused on the greater good of union with God for yourself, your spouse, and your children is the only way to make your plans for your life harmonious with God the Father's plan of loving goodness.

❖ Make frequent acts of faith to increase your trust in God. Say, "Lord, I believe; help my unbelief!" or simply "Jesus, I trust in you!"

❖ Practice self-gift toward your spouse in multiple ways every day. Try doing something your spouse would especially appreciate: unloading the dishwasher without being asked or making a point of greeting him when he comes home.

❖ Practice tenderness. Can you enlarge your expressive vocabulary? How else other than sex can you express tenderness for your spouse? Try to express affection for your spouse in one new, non-sexual way every day.

Virtuous practice involves outward actions such as these. But it also involves what our Lord calls the "heart": "But I say to you that everyone who looks at a woman with lust has already committed adultery with her in his heart" (Mt 5:28). A person who has already lived unchastely has to be particularly attentive to habits of the heart, which are the source of our actions. I cannot expect to move from simply saying "no" to bad sex to saying "yes" to self-giving love (chastity) without new habits of the heart.

To what should I be alert when it comes to my heart? Here are some questions that might be helpful:

❖ Am I driven by insecurity that leads me to seek out people who want to use others and be used sexually? Women, do you feel as though you have little worth if you are not sexually active? Men, do you feel insufficiently manly if you are not sexually active?

❖ Am I always sizing up the opposite sex as potential romantic or sexual partners to satisfy my emotional and physical needs, or do I view them first as persons dreamed up by the Father before the foundation of the world to be a unique saint?

❖ If married, am I becoming unduly emotionally attached to someone of the opposite sex who is not my spouse? Here are some good guidelines: Do I feel as though I need to hide the significance of this relationship from my spouse? Do I think about spending time with this person more than with my spouse?

Sometimes two spouses have a simultaneous conversion to secondary fruitfulness after spending time exploring it together. But what if your spouse is lagging behind in accepting this teaching? The one-flesh nature of the marital union makes this a delicate issue to negotiate. Actions like a sexual strike until one's spouse agrees with Catholic teaching are problematic; conversely, so is forcing bad sex.[1] The believer should begin with gently finding ways to educate his or her spouse concerning the reasons for Church teaching. Ask the Holy Spirit for persuasive words. If the relationship is already mature enough to allow for honest and open communication, this is certainly the time for it! Perhaps this book or another explanation of Church teaching would be helpful.

If the other spouse is too hostile to the idea of NFP to have a calm discussion, then prayer and example are the best approach. Saint Monica is a patron saint of women (and men) in such difficult situations. What ultimately persuades is not just reasonable argumentation but also love. You, the believing spouse, should focus not on what you cannot do: fixing your spouse—but on what you can do, through the grace of God: growing in holiness yourself. Begin by practicing spousal self-gift in other ways. If you become holier, this will automatically improve your marriage. The rest you must leave up to God.

These ideas are just suggested starting points. Any action that makes you a better person and a better spouse will make easier your living in accord with God the Father's plan for your fertility.

CONCLUSION

From Fear to Trust

This book began with an observation that fear drives our contraceptive culture even more than sexual urges do. We fear what we might have to give up if we are receptive to reality, so we become egoists instead. We fear the Father's plan of loving goodness for our lives, so we try to create our own plan from scratch. We fear *losing control*, so we cling to *birth control*.

Scripture teaches us that the antidote for fear is *love*. "Perfect love casts out fear" (1 Jn 4:18). If we are afraid, it is because we do not love enough. Before he became pope, John Paul II wrote that, rather than fearing limitations on our freedom, true love goes hand in hand with such limitations in the service of a much greater freedom: the freedom to love.

> Love consists in a commitment of freedom, because, after all, love is self-giving, and to give oneself means precisely to limit one's freedom on account of the other person. The limitation of one's own freedom would be something negative and unpleasant, but love makes it something positive, joyful, and creative. Freedom is for love.[1]

Our exemplar of fearless, loving freedom is Mary. At the moment of the Annunciation, the angel Gabriel approaches her and asks her if she will consent to bear the Son of God. She asks, "How can this be, since I am a virgin?" He answers, "The Holy Spirit will come upon you, and the power of the Most High will overshadow you" (Lk 1:34–35). Am I the only reader who has felt that Gabriel doesn't provide all the relevant data? In Mary's situation, I would have had lots of further questions: What exactly is this going to entail? What about Joseph? Can I have a little time to think about it? But Mary, acting not out of fear but out of her deep and trusting love for God, simply says *fiat*, let it be done unto me according to your Word. And Mary is our Mother in the spiritual life, who communicates her receptivity to us.

Very often in life, we must proceed without having all the answers. This is no accident. It is deliberate on God the Father's part: He wants us to learn to trust. We are called to trust especially when it comes to our fertility, because it is about our future, which is a treasure stored in the Father's invisible country of delight. May our response to our heavenly Father's loving will for us in this, as in all areas of our life, be that of Mary's love: *fiat*. Let it be done unto me according to your Word.

Notes

Chapter Two

1. Kevin Drum, "Catholics Do Not Have a Deep Moral Objection to Birth Control," *Mother Jones*, February 7, 2012, http://www.motherjones.com/kevin-drum/2012/02/catholics-do-not-have-moral-objection-contraception.

2. Daniel Maguire, "The Moderate Roman Catholic Position on Contraception and Abortion," *The Religious Consultation on Population Reproductive Health and Ethics*, http://www.religiousconsultation.org/News_Tracker/moderate_RC_position_on_contraception_abortion.htm.

3. Robert G. Hoyt, ed., "Majority Report of the Papal Commission," ch. 3, *The Birth Control Debate* (Kansas City: National Catholic Reporter, 1968).

4. Ibid., ch. 2.

5. Karalen L. Morthole, "My Take: Why I Am a Catholic for Contraception," *CNN*, February 10th, 2012, http://religion.blogs.cnn.com/2012/02/10/my-take-why-im-a-catholic-for-contraception/.

Chapter Three

1. Dr. Janet Smith, "Contraception: Why Not?" http://www.janetsmith.excerptsofinri.com/.

2. For a comparison of NaProTECHNOLOGY with in vitro fertilization (IVF) in treating infertility, see "Infertility," NaPro Technology.com, http://www.naprotechnology.com/infertility.htm. NaProTECHNOLOGY's success in treating infertility due to endometriosis is 56.7 percent, for example, while IVF's success rate is 21.2 percent. IVF's success rate for all couples is less than 30 percent in achieving pregnancy and less than 23 percent for achieving a live birth: "Infertility and In Vitro Fertilization," WebMD.com, http://www.webmd.com/infertility-and-reproduction/guide/in-vitro-fertilization?page=2. Why is NaProTECHNOLOGY so superior to IVF? NaProTECHNOLOGY monitors the woman's cycle to determine the underlying problem that is causing the infertility, and then aims to treat the problem. IVF is a technological run-around: it simply brings together sperm and egg in a laboratory environment and then inserts the fertilized egg (or eggs) into the womb. Nothing has been treated. For more, see Katie Elrod and Paul Carpentier, "The Church's Best Kept Secret: Church Teaching on Infertility Treatment," in *Women, Sex, and the Church*, ed. Erika Bachiochi (Boston: Pauline Books & Media, 2010), 121–42; Jean Dimech-Juchniewicz, *Facing Infertility: A Catholic Approach* (Boston: Pauline Books & Media, 2012); and Carmen Santamaria and Angeligue Ruhi-Lopez, *The Infertility Companion for Catholics* (Notre Dame, IN: Ave Maria Press, 2012).

Chapter Seven

1. See Bill Cosby, *To Russell, My Brother, Whom I Slept With*, Track 4, "The Apple." Released by Warner Bros / Wea on April 28, 1998.

2. The Association of Reproductive Health Professionals states that the perfect-use failure rate of the sympto-thermal method of NFP is 0.4 percent, while it is 0.3 percent for the combined and the

progestin-only birth-control pills: "Choosing a Birth Control Method: Contraceptive Failure Rates: Table," Association of Reproductive Health Professionals, Sept. 2011, http://www.arhp. org/Publications-and-Resources/Quick-Reference-Guide-for-Clinicians/choosing/failure-rates-table.

3. Ibid.

4. "Facts on Induced Abortion in the United States," Guttmacher Institute, Aug. 2011, http://www.guttmacher.org/pubs/fb_induced_abortion.html.

Chapter Eight

1. See, e.g., Mercedes Arzú Wilson, "The Practice of Natural Family Planning Versus the Use of Artificial Birth Control: Family, Sexual, and Moral Issues," *Catholic Social Science Review* 7 (November 2002) (showing a 0.2 percent divorce rate among NFP couples). Couple to Couple League's studies of NFP couples indicate up to a 4 percent divorce rate in "Marital Duration and Natural Family Planning," http://web.archive.org/web/20070818184432/http://ccli.org/nfp/marriage/maritalduration.php.

Chapter Nine

1. The United States Supreme Court decision used precisely this logic to uphold legal abortion on demand: "At the heart of liberty is the right to define one's own concept of existence, of meaning, of the universe, and of the mystery of human life." *Planned Parenthood of Southeastern PA vs. Casey*, 505 U.S. 833 (1992).

2. Pope Paul VI, *Humanae Vitae: A Challenge to Love*, trans. Janet E. Smith (New Hope, KY: New Hope Publications, 1987), no. 17.

3. Ibid.

4. Ibid.

5. Frederick Osborn, "Notes on 'Paradigms or Public Relations': The Case of Social Biology," 2, January 25, 1974, cited in Angela

Franks, *Margaret Sanger's Eugenic Legacy: The Control of Female Fertility* (Jefferson, N.C.: McFarland, 2005), 83.

6. Margaret Sanger, *Woman and the New Race* (NY: Blue Ribbon Books, 1920), 229.

7. Jonas B. Robitscher, ed., *Eugenic Sterilization* (Springfield, IL: Charles C. Thomas, 1973), 118–19.

8. Paul Ehrlich, *The Population Bomb* (NY: Ballantine, 1968), 15.

9. "The World's Vanishing Children," Population Research Institute, http://www.pop.org/.

10. Pope Paul VI, *Humanae Vitae*, no. 21.

Chapter Ten

1. Hoyt, Majority Papal Commission Report, ch. 3.

Chapter Eleven

1. "Strikingly, the proportion of men reporting three or more non-regular partners in the previous year fell from 15 to 3 percent between the 1989 and 1995 GPA surveys . . . . Such reported behavioral changes are consistent with the dominant AIDS prevention messages of Uganda's early response (i.e., 1986–1991), specifically: 'stick to one partner,' and the ubiquitous 'love faithfully' and 'zero-grazing' admonitions readily understood even by the many illiterate residents of this largely rural nation." Edward C. Green, et. al., "Uganda's HIV Prevention Success," *AIDS and Behavior* 10, no. 4 (July 2006): 335–46, doi: 10.1007/s10461-006-9073-y, reprinted by the National Center for Biotechnology Information, http://www.ncbi.nlm.nih.gov/pmc/articles/PMC154 4373/.

2. CDC, "Teenagers in the United States: Sexual Activity, Contraceptive Use, and Childbearing, National Survey of Family Growth, 2006–2008," *Vital and Health Statistics* 23, no. 30 (June 2012): 10, http://www.cdc.gov/nchs/data/series/sr_23/sr23_030.pdf. According to the CDC, 95 percent of teenagers had used the condom, while 58 percent had used withdrawal, and 55 percent the Pill.

3. Jason Deparle and Sabrina Tavernise, "Unwed Mothers Now a Majority Before Age of 30," *New York Times* (February 18, 2012), A1.

4. The articles on the topic are numerous. See, among others: R. Haveman, B. Wolfe, and K. Pence, "Intergenerational effects of nonmarital and early childbearing," in *Out of Wedlock: Causes and Consequences of Nonmarital Fertility*, eds. L. L. Wu and B. Wolfe (New York: Russell Sage Foundation, 2001); D. Demo and M. Cox, "Families with Young Children: A Review of Research in the 1990s," *Journal of Marriage and the Family* 62, no. 4 (Nov. 2000): 876-895; S. McLanahan and G. Sandefur, *Growing up with a Single Parent: What Hurts, What Helps* (Cambridge: Harvard University Press, 2004); Marcia Carlson and Mary Corcoran, "Family Structure and Children's Behavioral and Cognitive Outcomes," *Journal of Marriage and the Family* 63, no. 3 (Aug. 2001); and W. S. Aquilino, "The Life Course of Children Born to Unmarried Mothers: Childhood Living Arrangments and Young Adult Outcomes," *Journal of Marriage and the Family* 58, no. 2 (May 1996): 293–310.

5. Deparle and Tavernise, "Unwed Mothers," A1.

6. Kathryn Edin and Maria Kefalas, *Promises I Can Keep: Why Poor Women Put Motherhood Before Marriage* (University of California Press, 2011), 6.

7. "Statutory Rape Crime Relationships Between Juveniles and Adults: A Review of Social Scientific Research," *Aggression and Violent Behavior* 12 (2007): 300–14.

8. See Robert T. Michael, "Why Did the U.S. Divorce Rate Double within a Decade?" *Research in Population Economics* 6 (1988): 367–99.

9. Edward Peters, "Contraception and Divorce: Insights from American annulment cases," Couple to Couple League Family Foundations (Nov.–Dec. 1998): 28–29, reprinted by CanonLaw.info, http://www.canonlaw.info/a_contraceptionand divorce.htm.

10. Ibid.

Chapter Twelve

1. See John Paul II, *Letter to Women* (Boston: Pauline Books & Media, 1995), nos. 10, 11.

2. See John Paul II, *Man and Woman He Created Them: A Theology of the Body*, trans. Michael Waldstein (Pauline Books & Media, 2006), par. 126–32.

3. See *Humanae Vitae*, no. 21.

Chapter Thirteen

1. *Catechism of the Catholic Church*, Vatican.va, http://www.vatican.va/archive/ENG0015/_INDEX.HTM.

2. CCC, no. 27.

3. See Pope Paul VI, Apostolic Exhortation *Evangelii Nuntiandi*, 1975, 41.

Chapter Fourteen

1. For more details on this subject, see Father Tad Pacholczyk, "To Give or Not to Give: That Is the Marital Question," *Colorado Catholic Herald*, Oct. 21, 2011, http://www.coloradocatholicherald.com/ArticleDetails/tabid/1249/ArticleID/123/MAKING-SENSE-OF-BIOETHICS-%E2%80%98To-Give-or-Not-to-Give%E2%80%99-That-Is-the-Marital-Question.aspx.

Conclusion

1. Karol Wojtyla, *Love and Responsibility*, trans. Grzegorz Ignatik (Boston: Pauline Books & Media, 2013), 117.

Further Reading

The works with an * indicate the most accessible books that are a good next step.

Church Documents

* *Catechism of the Catholic Church,* Second Edition. Washington, DC: United States Conference of Catholic Bishops, 2006.

* Pope John Paul II. *Letter to Women,* 1995, http://www.vatican.va/holy_father/john_paul_ii/letters/documents/hf_jp-ii_let_29061995_women_en.html.

———. Apostolic letter *Mulieris Dignitatem,* 1988, http://www.vatican.va/holy_father/john_paul_ii/apost_letters/1988/documents/hf_jp-ii_apl_19880815_mulieris-dignitatem_en.html.

———. *Man and Woman He Created Them: A Theology of the Body.* Translated by Michael Waldstein. Boston: Pauline Books & Media, 2006.

* Pope Paul VI. Encyclical *Humanae Vitae* as found in *Humanae Vitae: A Challenge to Love.* Translated by Janet E. Smith. New Hope, KY.: New Hope Publications, 1987.

Wojtyla, Karol/Pope John Paul II. *Love and Responsibility*. Translated by Grzegorz Ignatik. Boston: Pauline Books & Media, 2013.

Other Resources

* Doyle, Fletcher. *Natural Family Planning Blessed Our Marriage: 19 True Stories*. Saint Anthony Messenger Press, 2006.

* Eden, Dawn. *The Thrill of the Chaste: Finding Fulfillment While Keeping Your Clothes On*. Nashville: Thomas Nelson, 2006.

* Healy, Mary. *Men and Women Are from Eden: A Study Guide to John Paul II's Theology of the Body*. Cincinnati: Servant Books, 2006.

* Smith, Janet. "Contraception: Why Not?" CD/DVD. www.Janetesmith.com.

Smith, Janet, ed. *Why* Humanae Vitae *Was Right: A Reader*. San Francisco: Ignatius Press, 1993.

* Sri, Edward. *Men, Women, and the Mystery of Love: Practical Insights from John Paul II's Love and Responsibility*. Cincinnati: Servant Books, 2005.

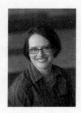

Author, speaker, professor, and television host, **Angela Franks, PhD**, describes herself as a theologian mom. With her husband, fellow theologian J. David Franks, she works to build a culture of life and love . . . starting within their own home. They raise their family, presently numbering six kids, in Boston, where she is the Director of Theology Programs for the Theological Institute for the New Evangelization at Saint John's Seminary.

Through her CatholicTV programs—*Christian Witness* and *The Future Depends on Love*—previous writings—*Margaret Sanger's Eugenic Legacy: The Control of Female Fertility* (McFarland, 2005) and a chapter on contraception in *Women, Sex, and the Church: A Case for Catholic Teaching* (Pauline Books & Media, 2010)—and her blogging at www.drsfranks.com, Dr. Franks witnesses to the gospel of love and life.

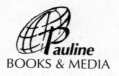

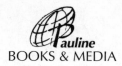

BOOKS & MEDIA

The Daughters of St. Paul operate book and media centers at the following addresses. Visit, call, or write the one nearest you today, or find us at www.pauline.org

CALIFORNIA

3908 Sepulveda Blvd, Culver City, CA 90230	310-397-8676
935 Brewster Avenue, Redwood City, CA 94063	650-369-4230
5945 Balboa Avenue, San Diego, CA 92111	858-565-9181

FLORIDA

145 S.W. 107th Avenue, Miami, FL 33174	305-559-6715

HAWAII

1143 Bishop Street, Honolulu, HI 96813	808-521-2731
Neighbor Islands call:	866-521-2731

ILLINOIS

172 North Michigan Avenue, Chicago, IL 60601	312-346-4228

LOUISIANA

4403 Veterans Memorial Blvd, Metairie, LA 70006	504-887-7631

MASSACHUSETTS

885 Providence Hwy, Dedham, MA 02026	781-326-5385

MISSOURI

9804 Watson Road, St. Louis, MO 63126	314-965-3512

NEW YORK

64 W. 38th Street, New York, NY 10018	212-754-1110

PENNSYLVANIA

Philadelphia—relocating	215-676-9494

SOUTH CAROLINA

243 King Street, Charleston, SC 29401	843-577-0175

VIRGINIA

1025 King Street, Alexandria, VA 22314	703-549-3806

CANADA

3022 Dufferin Street, Toronto, ON M6B 3T5	416-781-9131

¡También somos su fuente para libros,
videos y música en español!